T0006330

THE
CROHN'S DISEASE
COOKBOOK

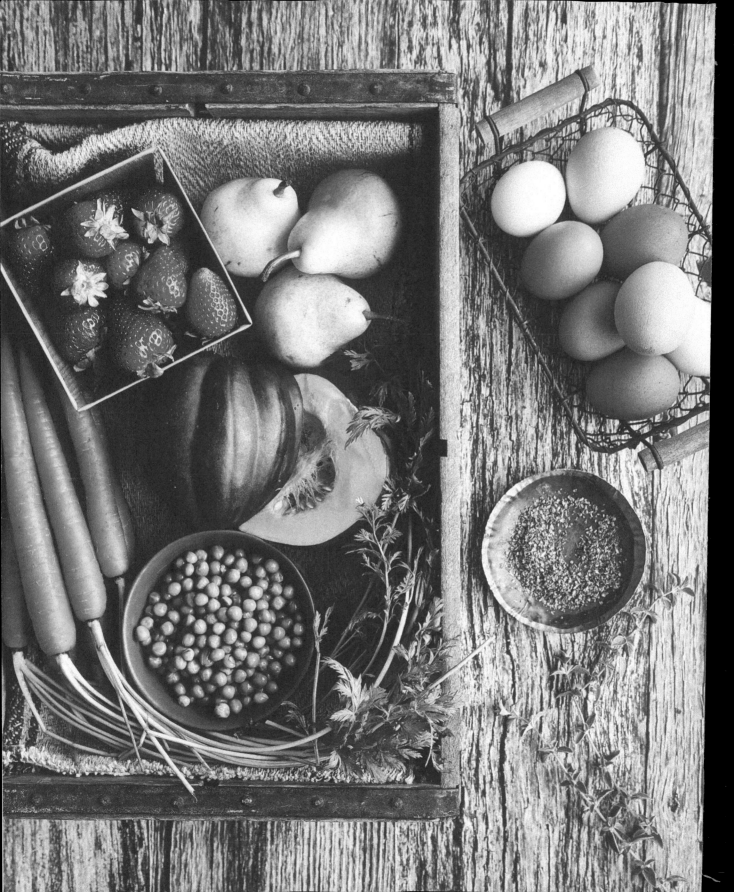

THE
CROHN'S DISEASE
COOKBOOK

100 RECIPES AND 2 WEEKS OF
MEAL PLANS TO RELIEVE SYMPTOMS

AMANDA FOOTE, RD

Photography by Hélène Dujardin

**ROCKRIDGE
PRESS**

Copyright © 2020 by Rockridge Press, Emeryville, California

No part of this publication may be reproduced, stored in a retrieval system, or transmitted in any form or by any means, electronic, mechanical, photocopying, recording, scanning, or otherwise, except as permitted under Sections 107 or 108 of the 1976 United States Copyright Act, without the prior written permission of the Publisher. Requests to the Publisher for permission should be addressed to the Permissions Department, Rockridge Press, 6005 Shellmound Street, Suite 175, Emeryville, CA 94608.

Limit of Liability/Disclaimer of Warranty: The Publisher and the author make no representations or warranties with respect to the accuracy or completeness of the contents of this work and specifically disclaim all warranties, including without limitation warranties of fitness for a particular purpose. No warranty may be created or extended by sales or promotional materials. The advice and strategies contained herein may not be suitable for every situation. This work is sold with the understanding that the publisher is not engaged in rendering medical, legal, or other professional advice or services. If professional assistance is required, the services of a competent professional person should be sought. Neither the Publisher nor the author shall be liable for damages arising herefrom. The fact that an individual, organization, or website is referred to in this work as a citation and/or potential source of further information does not mean that the author or the Publisher endorses the information the individual, organization, or website may provide or recommendations they/it may make. Further, readers should be aware that websites listed in this work may have changed or disappeared between when this work was written and when it is read.

For general information on our other products and services or to obtain technical support, please contact our Customer Care Department within the United States at (866) 744-2665, or outside the United States at (510) 253-0500.

Rockridge Press publishes its books in a variety of electronic and print formats. Some content that appears in print may not be available in electronic books, and vice versa.

TRADEMARKS: Rockridge Press and the Rockridge Press logo are trademarks or registered trademarks of Callisto Media Inc. and/or its affiliates, in the United States and other countries, and may not be used without written permission. All other trademarks are the property of their respective owners. Rockridge Press is not associated with any product or vendor mentioned in this book.

Interior and Cover Designer: Monica Cheng
Art Producer: Hannah Dickerson
Editor: Anne Lowrey
Production Editor: Andrew Yackira

Photography © Hélène Dujardin, 2020; food styling by Anna Hampton
Decorative patterns courtesy of Design Cuts, Shutterstock
Cover: Vegetable Paninis (p.96)

ISBN: Print 978-1-64739-313-7 | eBook 978-1-64739-314-4

R0

To anyone living with Crohn's disease,
you are not alone.

Contents

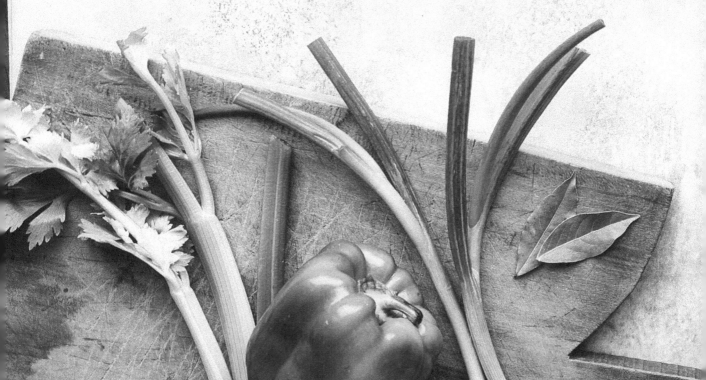

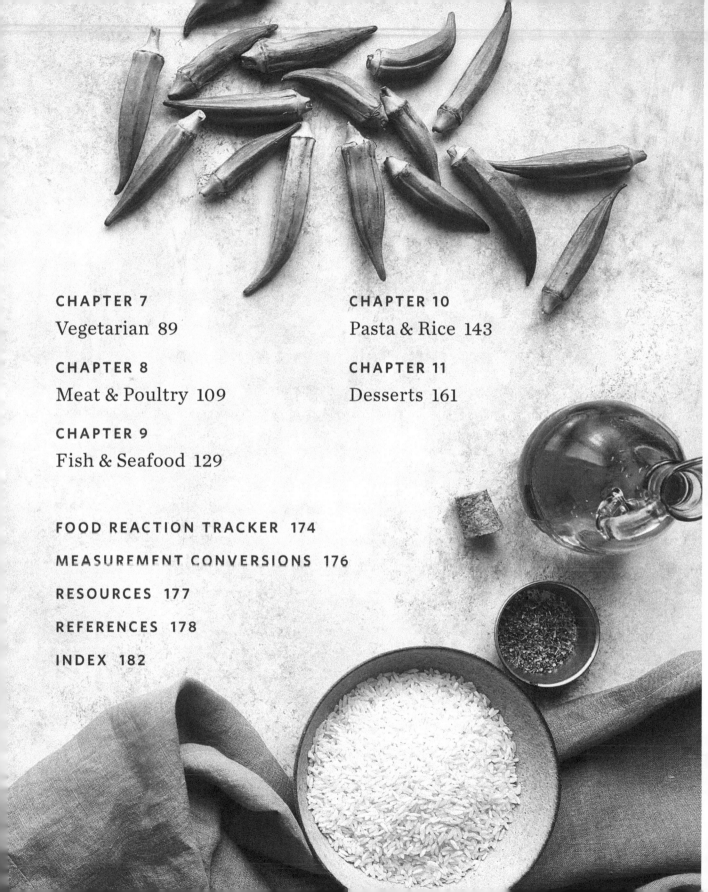

Introduction

My name is Amanda Foote. I am a registered dietitian, and I would like to thank you for welcoming me on your healing journey. I became a dietitian specifically to help people with food-related medical conditions such as Crohn's disease. While I do not have Crohn's, I do have food allergies and other chronic illnesses, so I understand and empathize with the feelings of frustration, confusion, and fear you may have concerning food. It is my professional and personal mission to help relieve those feelings, not only by providing helpful information, but also by bringing delicious, healthy, and comforting meals to your family table.

While everyone's health journey is different, I imagine that you, like many people with Crohn's disease, suffered for a long time before you were diagnosed. Sometimes, getting a proper diagnosis feels like a relief, because it validates your struggles, puts a name to your symptoms, and allows you to begin moving forward. On the other hand, getting a diagnosis of a chronic condition can be emotional and stressful because it will always be with you. Having worked with many clients in these circumstances, and having been through a similar situation myself, I sympathize with the challenges you are facing, and I am here to help.

Your life with Crohn's disease is completely unique. The diagnosis is a common umbrella, but the storms you weather are your own; every person's body and experience with the disease is different. Often, however, finding the right diet for your body can have a significant positive impact on the frequency and severity of your flare-ups and can increase the frequency or duration of remission.

Although there is no one way of eating that works for every person with Crohn's disease at all times, this book will help guide you through the challenges you are currently facing and teach you how to adopt the best diet and lifestyle for you, whether you are in a flare-up or in remission.

My goal with this book is to show you how choosing the right foods for your body can help you live more comfortably, feel more connected to your body, and regain a sense of control. As a dietitian, it is my ethical and professional responsibility to share recommendations that are backed by evidence-based science. You can rest assured that the guidance this book provides is scientifically sound, with a strong foundation in peer-reviewed studies and clinical trials.

You will find that the recipes are written with flexibility in mind so you can modify them to your specific sensitivities, nutritional needs, and preferences. In addition, they are easy to follow, have short ingredient lists, use simple cooking techniques, and include a wide variety of foods to provide bountiful nutrition and satisfaction.

One reason you might have sought out this book is that you have searched for healing from doctors, medications, and other treatments, but have yet to find relief from your symptoms. Food is a powerful tool that can have a big impact on your disease and symptoms, and you are in complete control of it.

The road to remission begins here!

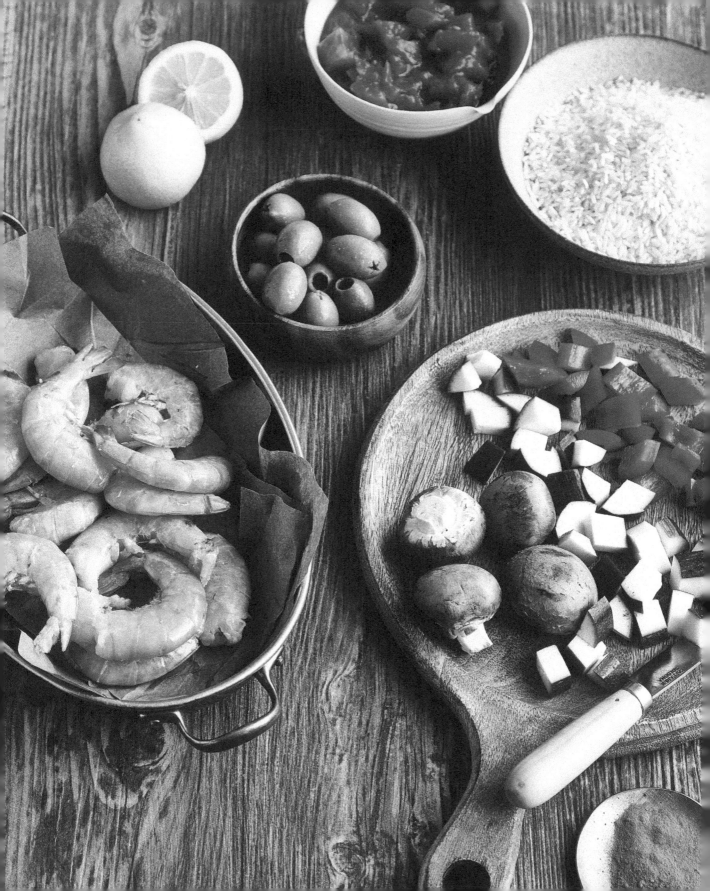

CHAPTER 1

The Crohn's Disease Diet Connection

In this chapter, I will cover what Crohn's disease is and what it looks like in daily life. I will also speak to how nutrition can help you heal, the role your mind can play in your healing, and how your doctor can help you. I'll explain how foods can affect your symptoms and share some recommendations for ensuring you are getting enough nutrients. These are the first steps in your journey toward feeling better.

What Is Crohn's Disease?

Inflammatory bowel disease (IBD) is a group of conditions that cause chronic inflammation in the digestive system. The two main types of IBD are Crohn's disease and ulcerative colitis.

Every instance of Crohn's disease is unique, since it affects every person differently. It can occur in any part of the gastrointestinal tract, but the most common type of Crohn's, called ileocolitis, occurs in the tail end of the small intestine and the beginning of the large intestine. Other forms of Crohn's are ileitis, which only affects the small intestine; gastroduodenal Crohn's, which affects the stomach; jejunoileitis, which affects only the beginning of the small intestine; and Crohn's colitis, which only affects the large intestine. No matter the type, Crohn's disease affects all layers of tissue and causes swelling, or inflammation, of the tissue that connects the intestine to the abdomen. In Crohn's disease, sections of healthy tissue in the intestines are separated by inflamed sections, which can produce flare-ups, or painful symptoms.

The term "inflammation" can be confusing because its presence in the body can be considered good or bad. Typically, when tissue gets irritated from infection or injury, an immune response is triggered to repair the damage, resulting in "good" inflammation that helps the body heal. The problem arises when this process is constant, and chronic inflammation develops.

The good news is that nutrition is an effective tool for resolving and preventing chronic inflammation, and this book will help you find the foods that work well for you, so you can feel better.

Causes

Crohn's disease is still a bit baffling to the medical community, because its causes are not well understood. One known cause of Crohn's disease is an overactive immune system. A normal immune system only attacks harmful microorganisms, but some people's immune systems attack harmless microorganisms as well. This is believed to be a cause of chronic inflammation in Crohn's disease.

Crohn's may also have genetic risk factors. Though many patients have immediate family members who also have Crohn's, many others have no familial history of IBD. Cultural background is not a cause of Crohn's disease; however, its prevalence has been shown to be higher in people of eastern European descent, including many Jewish people.

Where you live is not a direct cause of Crohn's disease, but the disease is more prevalent in urban areas of developed countries, particularly in northern climates. This may be because diets in urban areas of developed countries tend to be higher in processed and high-fat foods and lack healthy bacteria that can enrich the intestinal microbiome.

Living with Crohn's Disease: What We Know

For most people, the onset of Crohn's disease is in young adulthood, between the ages of 15 and 30, though it can occur in childhood or later in adulthood. Early symptoms may include unintentional weight loss, frequent abdominal pain or cramping, diarrhea, or blood in your stool.

To test you for Crohn's disease, your doctor will likely perform a physical exam, draw blood for blood tests, and ultimately send you to get an endoscopy. An endoscopy is a low-risk, nonsurgical procedure similar to a colonoscopy, where a tiny camera on a flexible tube is used to examine your digestive system for any damage that may have occurred from Crohn's inflammation.

Crohn's is a chronic and progressive condition, which means that you will have it for your lifetime and it will change over time. But this does not mean you will suffer for your entire life. Remission, or a stage in which Crohn's is not active in your body, is completely achievable. By listening to your body, working with your doctor, consulting with a dietitian, and using resources like this book, you can find the path to living your best life.

Symptoms

It is likely you have experienced a variety of symptoms in your digestive tract or elsewhere in your body as a result of Crohn's disease. These symptoms may vary or change over time, or over the course of a single flare-up. They may appear on a spectrum from sudden to gradual, or frequent to infrequent, and you may have long or short periods of remission, or time without symptoms. Because there can be so much variation with Crohn's, it is helpful to understand what you may experience.

As you begin your healing journey, the first step is to gain knowledge, and the second step is to raise your awareness. Being able to recognize, accurately track, and address your symptoms early will help you get on the road to healing more quickly.

Gastrointestinal symptoms may include:

- Abdominal pain
- Blood, pus, or mucus in the stool
- Constipation
- Cramping
- Diarrhea
- Feeling of incomplete defecation
- Increased urgency to defecate
- Pain around the anus
- Reduced appetite

Whole-body symptoms may include:

- Amenorrhea, for women (absence of menstrual period)
- Anemia
- Arthritis
- Eye inflammation
- Fatigue
- Fever
- Joint inflammation
- Kidney stones
- Liver inflammation
- Mouth sores
- Osteoporosis
- Rashes
- Skin inflammation
- Unintentional weight loss

In this book, I will discuss in detail how lifestyle, stress management, and, most of all, food can help alleviate your symptoms. With time, you will learn the specific foods and habits that can help you feel better, and you will be able to better manage the symptoms that are specific to your body. I will make suggestions with the aim of helping, but the most important thing is to listen to your own body and learn how to respond to it, so you can feel your best as often as possible.

ULCERATIVE COLITIS

If you are living with ulcerative colitis, which is related to but different from Crohn's, this book can still help you. While Crohn's disease causes patches of inflammation in the small intestine and sometimes the large intestine, ulcerative colitis is limited to the large intestine, or colon. The nutrition guidance in this book can also help soothe symptoms of ulcerative colitis.

Overlapping recommendations specific to ulcerative colitis include avoiding greasy foods, limiting dairy, avoiding foods that cause gas and bloating, eating small, frequent meals, staying hydrated, and modifying fiber intake to meet your individual needs.

Each recipe that I crafted for Crohn's disease, whether for remission or flares, is also suitable for ulcerative colitis. Look for labels that can be helpful to you, like **DAIRY-FREE, LOW FIBER, LOW FODMAP,** and **LOW FAT**. Use the recipes in this book to help you find the foods that work best for your unique experience with IBD.

Crohn's Disease Day-to-Day

There are ways to manage Crohn's disease so that you can live a happy and full life. One of the best ways to do so is by paying attention to what you eat on a daily basis. Food can be a source of healing, not only by providing nourishment and comfort, but also as medicine.

Nurturing through Nutrition

When you are suffering, you might feel like you have little control. Yet, nutrition is a choice you *do* have control over; your food choices are a powerful tool in your journey to living well with Crohn's disease.

Although you will most likely use a combination of treatments for your symptoms, one of the best ways to prevent flare-ups and feel better in your daily life is to consistently eat nutritious foods that work for your unique digestive system.

Every diet, including one for Crohn's, should include protein, healthy fats, vitamins, and minerals. A Crohn's nutrition plan focuses on B vitamins, especially folate, vitamins C, D, and K, calcium, selenium, and zinc, which the recipes in this book abundantly provide. It is particularly important that your daily meals include these because it is often harder for your body to absorb nutrients.

Inflammation in the small intestine can cause malabsorption of nutrients, while inflammation in the large intestine can inhibit the absorption of water and electrolytes. It is important to pay attention to—without being afraid of—any signs of malnutrition. Watch for symptoms like fatigue, light-headedness, paleness, numbness, tingling, bruising, bone or muscle pain, hair loss, muscle cramping or spasms, appetite loss, and change in sense of taste or smell. It is important that you call your doctor if you notice these symptoms so they can help you begin correcting any deficiencies as soon as possible.

The goal of this book is to give you the tools you need to feel better and enjoy your food again. A balanced, nutrient-filled diet that is restorative, protective, and alleviates your symptoms is a great place to start.

RECOMMENDED SUPPLEMENTS

If you are having a lot of flare-ups or are experiencing deficiencies, you can use vitamin and mineral supplements to enhance your diet. Supplements you might want to consider include:

- B_6
- B_{12}
- Calcium
- Folic acid (a synthetic form of folate found in supplements)
- Iron
- Magnesium
- Omega-3 fatty acids
- Selenium
- Vitamin D
- Vitamin K
- Zinc

Taking a multivitamin is a great place to start before buying individual supplements, unless your doctor or dietitian advises otherwise.

Food itself is fuel, so focusing on getting vitamins through your food is most efficient and may minimize your need for supplements. Here are my tips:

- Include protein with every meal, if your body tolerates it. Meat, fish, dairy, eggs, legumes, and tofu provide B_6, B_{12}, iron, magnesium, omega-3s, selenium, vitamin D, and zinc. If you do not eat meat, plant-based protein sources include tofu, creamy nut and seed butters, beans, and peas.

- Dairy products, if tolerated, are a source of B_{12}, calcium, vitamin D, and zinc. Most dairy products, including lactose-free dairy products, are enriched with vitamin D, but check the label to make sure. If you do not eat dairy, nondairy milks and yogurts are also rich in these nutrients.

- Most grains are a good source of vitamins and minerals. Refined grains are lower in vitamins and minerals than whole grains, but cereals are almost always fortified with B vitamins, folic acid, and iron. Oats, especially rolled oats, are typically easy on the stomach and are an excellent source of vitamins and minerals.

- Low-fiber fruits like melons and bananas contain a wide variety of vitamins and minerals.

- Vegetables are excellent sources of vitamins and minerals, and they tend to be easier on the digestive system when well cooked, because cooking breaks down the fiber. Squash and spinach are nutrient powerhouses that contain vitamin K, calcium, and magnesium.

- Potatoes and sweet potatoes are easily digested and are excellent sources of iron, selenium, and magnesium. They also contain calcium, folic acid, and zinc.

Minding Your Body

An important first step in managing Crohn's disease is to learn how to listen to your body. Examples of listening to your body include noticing that you are a little cranky and asking yourself if you are hungry, or giving yourself permission to take a break when you feel more tired than usual. As you develop this skill, you will learn to recognize your own Crohn's-related symptoms, triggers, and warning signs and be able to respond with proactive interventions sooner.

The mind-body connection, which links our thoughts and emotions to how our body feels, and vice versa, is an ever-growing area of interest and research. There is a strong link between the gut and the brain. Sayings like "go with your gut" and "I have a gut feeling" are not just clichés. The enteric nervous system in our gastrointestinal tract contains millions of nerve cells that communicate with the brain.

The relationship between stress and inflammation provides a good example of the mind-body connection. Stress increases the levels of hormones and chemicals that cause inflammation in the body, which can increase your mental stress level, creating a cycle of chronic stress and inflammation. But, happily, the opposite is also true: Reducing stress can do wonders for reducing the inflammation linked to your Crohn's symptoms. If you start to notice a flare-up, take steps to reduce stress and focus on self-care.

One way to practice self-care is through mindfulness, a practice of focusing on the emotions, thoughts, and physical sensations you are experiencing in the moment. It can be as simple as sitting in a comfortable spot and taking an inventory of what you are experiencing. You can ask yourself, "What does the temperature of the air feel like on my skin?" or "What sensations am I feeling in my body?" or "What do I smell?" These simple questions bring your consciousness into a state of mindful awareness that can be incredibly relaxing.

When you are feeling overwhelmed or anxious, take a moment to practice mindfulness by doing one of the following:

- Take some time to relax and breathe. Have a cool drink of water and give yourself permission to slow down and do whatever your mind and body need.

- Take note of a few things you feel grateful for; gratitude can completely reframe your state of mind.

- Get a change of scenery. Step outside and focus on how the sun or the air feels on your face.

- Listen to a song you enjoy, or one that relaxes you.

- Take a short walk or do some comfortable, calming exercise.

Medication

The chart on pages 10 through 12 includes the most commonly prescribed medications and supplements. Bookmark these pages and refer to them anytime you have a new prescription or are wondering how your medication works, what side effects you might experience, and how it will affect your diet. Information is power, so use this table to empower yourself with knowledge.

CONVERSATIONS TO HAVE WITH YOUR DOCTOR

First, listen to your body, then discuss what you know about yourself and your symptoms with your doctor. Medical professionals are invaluable partners in your journey to remission. The following questions will help you get the most out of your next doctor's appointment.

- What parts of my bowel are affected by IBD, and what nutrients are typically absorbed in this location?
- How can I tell if a food is a trigger?
- How can I tell if I am in a flare-up?
- What can I eat to prevent flare-ups?
- What deficiencies should I be mindful of, and what should I eat to avoid deficiencies?
- Do I need to take any supplements?
- How can I tell if I am in remission? What can I eat during remission to replenish my nutrient stores?
- What can I do to manage stress? What kinds of exercise can I do that will not aggravate my symptoms?
- What side effects could my medications cause? What can I do to reduce any discomfort?
- What deficiencies could my medications cause? Will I need to take a supplement?
- Should I eat foods that contain probiotics? Do I need to take a prebiotic or probiotic supplement?

MEDICATION	CLASS	PURPOSE	SIDE EFFECTS & NUTRIENT CHALLENGES
Corticosteroids	Anti-inflammatory	Short-term reduction of inflammation to improve symptoms or trigger remission	• Excess sodium can cause water retention • Bone weakness will require calcium and vitamin D supplementation • Focus on getting adequate protein and potassium
Aminosalicylates	Anti-inflammatory	Reduce inflammation in the intestines	• Nausea, vomiting, abdominal pain, cramping, loss of appetite • Eat foods you can tolerate to ensure adequate intake and nutrition
Azathioprine and mercaptopurine	Immunosuppressant	Suppress overactive immune system	• Nausea, vomiting, diarrhea, loss of appetite, feeling full early, fever, fatigue • Eat foods you can tolerate to ensure adequate intake and nutrition

MEDICATION	CLASS	PURPOSE	SIDE EFFECTS & NUTRIENT CHALLENGES
Infliximab, adalimumab, and certolizumab	Immunosuppressant (TNF inhibitor or biologics)	Neutralize TNF (tumor necrosis factor), an immune system protein	• Stomach pain, fatigue, dizziness, nausea, diarrhea, constipation • Eat foods you can tolerate to ensure adequate intake and nutrition • Avoid undercooked eggs and meats, unpasteurized dairy, and soft cheeses
Methotrexate	Immunosuppressant	Suppress immune response (often used if you have not responded to other treatments)	• Stomach pain, nausea, vomiting, diarrhea, fatigue, mouth sores • Take a folic acid supplement to reduce side effects • Avoid alcohol
Natalizumab and vedolizumab	Immunosuppressant	Stop integrins (immune system molecules) from binding to the intestinal lining	• Nausea, stomach pain, diarrhea, severe headache, fever, altered mental state • Eat foods you can tolerate to ensure adequate intake and nutrition
Ustekinumab	Immunosuppressant	Block inflammatory agents that cause chronic inflammation in the GI tract	• Diarrhea, fatigue, rash, headache • Eat foods you can tolerate to ensure adequate intake and nutrition

MEDICATION	PURPOSE	SIDE EFFECTS & NUTRIENT CHALLENGES
Antibiotics	Reduce harmful bacteria or infection, which can help heal abscesses and fistulas	• Nausea, vomiting, diarrhea, vomiting, heartburn, stomach cramping, loss of appetite • Avoid dairy products for three hours after dosing, but the live cultures in yogurt can prevent yeast infections while on antibiotics • Avoid grapefruit and grapefruit juice • Consider a B_{12} supplement with frequent antibiotic use • May interact with iron supplements
Antidiarrheal agents	Reduce diarrhea	• Eat foods you can tolerate to ensure adequate intake and nutrition
Acetaminophen	Relieve pain	• Avoid grapefruit and grapefruit juice
Iron supplement	Replenish iron stores if you have bleeding	• Constipation, stomach pain, nausea, vomiting • Eating oatmeal and cooked vegetables can help settle your stomach • May interact with antibiotics
B_{12} supplement	Correct any B_{12} deficiency, which can impair nerve function	• Folic acid supplements interfere with B_{12} supplements
Calcium and vitamin D supplements	Prevent osteoporosis related to Crohn's disease	• Nausea, vomiting, constipation, bloating • Caffeine can impair absorption

How Food Affects Symptoms

Each person with Crohn's disease has their own unique relationship with food. Foods that are well tolerated for some people may trigger symptoms in others. For that reason, I encourage you to use the Food Reaction Tracker (page 174) to find your own safest foods and trigger foods so you can tailor your diet to your individual needs. Working with a dietitian is also a great way to manage this process.

Because this book is written for anyone with Crohn's disease, we will be talking about diet commonalities and generalizations, which you can then apply to your body to make them work for you.

To begin with, a person with Crohn's disease should generally avoid foods that are known to trigger flare-ups, including:

Fatty and greasy foods, such as fried foods, butter, mayonnaise, and red meat

Caffeinated foods, such as coffee, sodas, and tea

Foods that cause gas and bloating, such as cruciferous vegetables (broccoli, brussels sprouts, cabbage), beans, legumes, and lentils

Dairy products, which can cause gas for many people but can cause more uncomfortable symptoms for people with lactose intolerance

High-fiber foods, such as whole grains, raw fruits, and vegetables

Foods that may not get fully digested and could become lodged in the intestines, such as corn, nuts, and seeds

Spicy foods

Alcohol

What about food allergies? Crohn's disease does not cause food intolerances or food allergies, but it can be exacerbated by them. Food sensitivities, on the other hand, are much more common in people with Crohn's disease.

Any of the types of foods listed above can cause sensitivities or flare-ups. To manage these food sensitivities, you may need to limit or eliminate certain foods. The following are ways you adjust your diet to address common sensitivities:

Lactose Intolerance

A diet for lactose intolerance limits or excludes foods that contain lactose. These include milk (skim, 1%, 2%, whole, buttermilk), cream (heavy cream, sweet cream, whipping cream, half-and-half, sour cream), butter (salted, unsalted, clarified, ghee), cheese (solid, cream cheese, cottage cheese), yogurt, custard, pudding, and ice cream, as well as all products that are made with these ingredients. Common foods to look out for include baked goods (bread, biscuits, buns, rolls, cakes, cookies), pancakes, waffles, crackers, flavored chips, and chocolate. Lactose can be hidden in an ingredients list, but typically, a label will say CONTAINS MILK if it contains lactose. Other ingredients to look for on a label include casein, caseinates, and whey.

A lactose-free diet can include all other food groups, including meat, grains, fruit, and vegetables. It is worth noting that you can find lactose-free versions of many dairy products, including milk, yogurt, sour cream, and cream cheese.

Low-Fiber or Low-Residue Foods

A low-fiber or low-residue diet aims to lower fiber in the diet to reduce stools and give the intestines some rest.

High-fiber foods to avoid include whole grains (such as wheat, bran, and rye), raw fruits and vegetables (especially with the skin on), beans, lentils, leafy green vegetables, popcorn, whole nuts, seeds, and corn.

Foods to include while eating low-residue include white bread, white pasta, white rice, skinless cooked vegetables, certain fruits (like bananas and melons), eggs, fish, chicken, and dairy products. It may seem contradictory to include dairy products, but you should only include dairy products if you are not lactose intolerant and they are not a trigger for you. Just because dairy is low residue does not mean it is suitable for every Crohn's diet.

Low-FODMAP Diet

FODMAP is an acronym that stands for "fermentable oligosaccharides, disaccharides, monosaccharides, and polyols." In other words:

Fructose: found in table sugar, fruits, vegetables (only fruits and vegetables with excess fructose are considered high FODMAP), high-fructose corn syrup, honey, and fruit juice

Lactose: found in dairy products

Fructans: found in grains, including wheat, bran, and rye (including alcohols made from these grains), as well as garlic and onion

Galactans: found in legumes like beans and peas

Polyols: sugar alcohols used as sweeteners

A low-FODMAP diet is more of a diagnostic tool than a long-term diet. It can, at first, seem incredibly restrictive, but remember that the goal of the FODMAP diet is not to eliminate all foods from your diet forever, but rather to determine which particular FODMAPs you are sensitive to and only eliminate those from your diet for the long term. Then, you can reintroduce foods you tolerate well.

In stage one, you should avoid all high-FODMAP foods for at least three weeks. In stage two, you begin reintroducing one high-FODMAP food at a time, for three days each, to test whether you can tolerate the food well or if it triggers symptoms. In stage three, you reintroduce the foods that worked well for you, and this becomes your ongoing diet.

We will discuss more about elimination diets, as well as an overall anti-inflammatory diet for remission periods, in the next chapter.

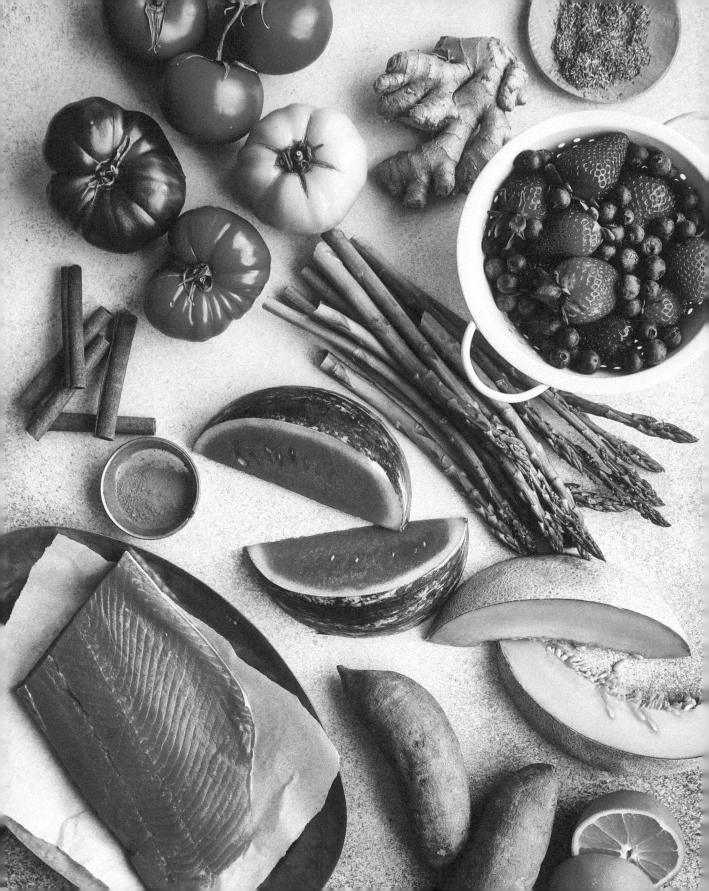

CHAPTER 2

Food Guidance for Crohn's Disease

Now that you have some background on Crohn's disease, you can start making a personal game plan for feeling better. This chapter will discuss in depth what, how, and when to eat in a way that best suits your body. I'll touch upon the best foods to eat overall, as well as how to tailor your eating when experiencing a flare-up. You will also learn more about your triggers, tracking your symptoms, stocking an IBD-friendly kitchen, and how to use the recipes in this book.

An Anti-Inflammatory Diet

Crohn's disease is often defined by inflammation in the body, and inflammation can aggravate symptoms by triggering a flare-up. One of the best ways to fight inflammation is to adopt an anti-inflammatory diet.

Anti-inflammatory foods are great multitaskers for your health, because they not only nourish your body, but also help soothe your system. Use these helpful guidelines for adding more anti-inflammatory foods to your diet:

- Test anti-inflammatory foods one by one to ensure they are gentle on your system.

- If a food is healing for you, feel free to eat it in abundance. The anti-inflammatory foods discussed in this chapter will add both nutrients and flavor to your diet.

- Enjoy the flavor of your food. The recipes in this book introduce delicious flavor combinations that are also anti-inflammatory. Mix and match them to get some variety.

Many powerful anti-inflammatory foods are recommended when eating for Crohn's, as they tend to be highly protective rather than triggering. I recommend including the following foods to reduce inflammation and prevent flare-ups.

10 ANTI-INFLAMMATORY POWER FOODS

1. Turmeric
2. Ginger
3. Cinnamon
4. Olive oil
5. Fatty fish
6. Berries and citrus fruits (or juice, for less fiber)
7. Tomato
8. Creamy nut or seed butters
9. Garlic
10. Dark chocolate (many dark chocolates are dairy-free)

So many of us have difficulty drinking enough water. Life gets busy. Sometimes a day goes by and you find that you've barely touched that water bottle you packed. But hydration is key to fighting inflammation, because your kidneys, which filter toxins from your blood, need plenty of water to function properly.

Dehydration can cause your cells to release chemicals in the body that create inflammation. Follow these helpful tips for watching hydration levels:

- Note how often and how much you are urinating. If you are urinating less than usual, you might be dehydrated. Also note the color of your urine. When you are well hydrated, your urine should be clearer. (Note: this can be tricky if you are taking B vitamin supplements, because they tend to color urine bright yellow or orange.)

- Notice if you are having more headaches. Dehydration can cause headaches or migraines.

- Check in with yourself to determine if you are more tired or sleepy than usual. Although fatigue is common with Crohn's disease, especially during flare-ups, a general feeling of tiredness can be a sign of dehydration.

A general anti-inflammatory diet is best for the remission periods of Crohn's, to further protect from flare-ups. However, these principles can also be followed during flare-ups. If anti-inflammatory foods are effective for you, they are safe to incorporate into your daily meals, regardless of whether you are in remission or in a flare-up.

MANAGING CROHN'S DISEASE: WHAT TO EAT AT A GLANCE

When managing Crohn's disease, there are some foods you should avoid altogether, some you should limit, and some that are healing and should be eaten in abundance. The goal is to lessen overall symptoms and reduce flare-ups while ▸

FOODS TO ENJOY

- Avocado
- Banana
- Berries (or berry juice)
- Cinnamon
- Citrus fruits (or citrus juice)
- Cooked vegetables
- Creamy nut and seed butters
- Dairy-free dark chocolate
- Fatty fish
- Garlic (if tolerated)
- Ginger
- Hot and cold cereals
- Lactose-free or regular dairy products (if tolerated)
- Meat you can tolerate, such as chicken or lean cuts of beef or pork in smaller portions

- Melon
- Oats
- Olive oil and other plant-based cooking oils such as canola and vegetable oil
- Potatoes
- Skinless fruits and vegetables (preferably cooked)
- Squash
- Sweet potatoes
- Tofu
- Tomato
- Turmeric
- Water
- White grains like pasta, rice, and white bread

working to get as many nutrients as possible. Earmark this page for reference anytime you want an at-a-glance picture of what to eat to manage your Crohn's disease.

FOODS TO AVOID

- Alcohol
- Artificial sweeteners
- Beans, legumes, and lentils (unless well tolerated)
- Butter
- Caffeine
- Carbonated beverages
- Corn
- Cruciferous vegetables (broccoli, Brussels sprouts, cabbage)
- Dairy (if you are lactose intolerant or it is a trigger)
- Excess added sugar
- Grapefruit juice
- Greasy and fried foods
- High-fiber whole grains, fruits, and vegetables
- Mayonnaise
- Popcorn
- Red meat (unless well tolerated)
- Spicy foods
- Undercooked eggs and meats
- Unpasteurized dairy and soft cheeses
- Whole nuts and seeds

How and When to Eat

Many of us were raised on three large meals per day, with or without snacks between meals. This system may not be ideal if you have Crohn's disease, because you are giving your system large amounts of food to digest all at once. This can cause symptoms that increase your discomfort. Instead, it can be beneficial to eat four to six smaller meals over the course of the day. A sample day might include:

- Small breakfast
- Morning snack
- Small lunch
- Afternoon snack
- Small dinner
- Before-bed snack, if needed

Another problem is oversized portions. We can all be guilty of having eyes bigger than our stomachs and overloading our plates. This can leave us feeling uncomfortably full, which can be even more uncomfortable with Crohn's. Two effective strategies for avoiding oversized portions are:

1. Use salad plates instead of dinner plates.

2. Fill your plate with a small serving and get seconds after finishing it, instead of overfilling your plate and eating past fullness.

Chewing food more is also helpful for digestion, especially with Crohn's. The better you chew your food before swallowing, the less stress is placed on your esophagus, the less work your stomach has to do to break down and metabolize the food, and the less work your intestines have to do to digest the food and absorb the nutrients.

Food Considerations for Common Medications

While some people may be able to control their Crohn's through diet alone, others may find medications useful or necessary. As we discussed in chapter 1 (see pages 10 to 12), some medications have dietary implications. Some tips for modifying your diet on these different medications include:

CORTICOSTEROIDS

- Reduce sodium intake
- Supplement with calcium and vitamin D
- Include protein-rich foods when you can, including meat, dairy, beans, legumes, and soy, if you can tolerate them
- Include foods high in potassium like potatoes and bananas

AMINOSALICYLATES

- Focus on eating foods that you can tolerate; the goal is to eat enough for adequate nutrition, rather than focusing on specific foods

IMMUNOSUPPRESSANTS AND BIOLOGICS

- Like with aminosalicylates, focus on eating foods that you can tolerate
- Avoid undercooked eggs and meats, unpasteurized dairy, and soft cheeses
- Avoid alcohol
- You may need a folic acid supplement

ANTIBIOTICS

- Avoid dairy products for three hours after dosing, but the live cultures in yogurt can prevent yeast infections while on antibiotics
- Avoid grapefruit and grapefruit juice
- You may need a B_{12} supplement if you use antibiotics frequently

Food for Flare-ups

When you are in the middle of a flare-up, you need immediate relief. What you don't need is to be unsure about what is best for your system at that time. It will take listening to your own body to determine what works best for you, but here is some general guidance that can help you decode your body's needs:

Eat foods that you know are gentle on your system, including the 10 Healing Foods for Flare-ups (see page 25). During a flare-up, deciding which foods to eat can be stressful. A dietitian is a great resource for helping you craft a meal plan that gives you the best nutrition and comfort during flare-ups.

Avoid foods that you know are triggering or uncomfortable, including the 10 Foods to Avoid during Flare-ups (see page 25). In addition, using a system to track your food reactions, like the one on page 174, can be extremely helpful in identifying your specific triggers.

Choose foods that fight inflammation, including the 10 Anti-Inflammatory Power Foods (see page 18). Omega-3s and anti-inflammatory foods can add a boost of flavor to the gentle foods on your flare-up meal plan.

Stay hydrated! Drinking plenty of water makes digestion easier and will help prevent dehydration, which is often a concern during flare-ups. The general rule is to drink 64 ounces of water per day (or eight 8-ounce glasses). More exact guidance is based on your weight, with the average recommendation for Americans being 96 ounces per day for women and 125 ounces per day for men. Hydrating foods, such as safe fruits and vegetables, can also help you stay hydrated.

10 HEALING FOODS FOR FLARE-UPS

1. Hot and cold cereals, including oatmeal
2. White pasta
3. White rice
4. White bread
5. Potatoes
6. Bananas
7. Avocado
8. Poultry
9. Fish
10. Well-cooked, skinless vegetables

10 FOODS TO AVOID DURING FLARE-UPS

1. Whole nuts and seeds
2. Popcorn
3. High-fiber foods like whole grains, brown or wild rice, and raw fruits and vegetables with skins
4. Dairy
5. Spicy foods
6. High-fat foods like fried foods
7. Gas-causing foods like beans, legumes, and cruciferous vegetables
8. Red meat
9. Added sugars and artificial sweeteners
10. Caffeine, carbonation, and alcohol

FIGHTING FLARES

Food is not the only thing that can trigger flare-ups—stress also plays a big role. From a physiological perspective, acute and chronic stress raise hormones that cause inflammation, which can aggravate your Crohn's disease. From a practical perspective, when you are stressed, you likely are also not resting, eating well, or drinking enough water, all of which can trigger a flare-up.

Everyone experiences stress. We cannot completely eliminate it from our lives, but avoiding things that you know to be highly stressful can help you fight flare-ups. Overdoing activity or exercise while in a flare-up can exacerbate symptoms, because so much of your energy is going to healing your bowels, and the pain can be very draining.

Use these tips for adjusting your lifestyle once you have identified that you are in a flare-up.

Rest your body! Take more breaks during the day just to check in with yourself, breathe, and drink a glass of water.

Go to bed earlier. Give yourself the opportunity for a longer or better night's sleep.

Take a warm bath. A bath can soothe abdominal cramping, irritated perianal skin, and inflamed skin or rashes.

Practice mindfulness. Center your thoughts and calm your mind.

Inhale and exhale. Conscious breathing can help you relax. Many people also find calming scents to be effective at reducing stress. This does not have to mean essential oils in a fancy diffuser. An aroma that you grew up with and makes you happy, like vanilla or fresh oranges, works just as well.

Surround yourself with supportive, kind people. Ask these people for help with activities that are taxing for you, like grocery shopping or tidying the house.

Most importantly, **be kind to yourself.** Giving yourself grace during this time is essential. Crohn's disease is not your fault, you are doing your best, and your best IS enough!

Knowing Your Food Triggers

Anyone struggling with Crohn's disease may end up trying a variety of different approaches to discover what triggers flare-ups or irritates them most. One effective method for identifying food triggers is an elimination diet.

I recommend that you only eliminate one food (or a food grouping, like dairy or wheat) at a time. Eliminating multiple foods at a time makes it difficult to determine which food is bothering you. You might feel relief within days or a week, but it may take up to six weeks without a food to determine if it was a trigger for you.

You can follow an elimination diet for any food you suspect may be troubling you. You can begin by eliminating common triggers like gluten, dairy, red meat, or even individual triggers like particular fruits or vegetables.

Working around eliminated trigger foods is the basis for the labels you will find on the recipes in this book. You will find recipes that are gluten-free, dairy-free, low fat, low fiber, low FODMAP, and paleo.

A food-tracking chart is a helpful tool for you, your doctor, and your dietitian. Mindfully watch your symptoms in connection with certain foods for a week, and record your reactions. Information is power, and tracking your own reactions to individual foods is an excellent way to understand what triggers you.

Once you have identified your trigger foods, you will know what foods to avoid, which will help you prevent flare-ups. The best ways to avoid trigger foods in everyday life once you've identified them are to:

Read ingredient labels. All food products must list all ingredients and highlight major allergens—or, for you, sensitivities—at the end of the list. If a product contains milk, wheat, egg, peanuts, tree nuts, soy, fish, or shellfish, there will be a disclaimer at the end of the ingredients list that will say, for example, CONTAINS: WHEAT. Ingredient lists for restaurant meals must disclose major allergens as well. If you want to eat out and you cannot find the ingredient information online, a good strategy is to call ahead and ask. Or, when you go in person, ask to see an ingredient list and explain your dietary restrictions to a manager.

Prepare meals at home. The best way to ensure that trigger foods are completely avoided is to cook your own meals using whole ingredients. Prepackaged meals and convenience foods are likely to be full of trigger foods. By preparing your meals at home, you can have complete control over what foods go into your body.

The IBD-Friendly Kitchen

Stocking an IBD-friendly kitchen is an excellent way to make sure you have gentle foods on hand, which is especially important when you are feeling unwell. Having certain kitchen items well stocked, so you don't have to do lengthy shopping, will make cooking for Crohn's less stressful.

Pantry Essentials

Chances are that your pantry already has some favorite foods that you know work well for you. Perhaps your pantry also has some foods that taste good but are not gentle on your system. It can be helpful to refocus your pantry by eliminating highly processed convenience foods that likely contain triggers like dairy, wheat, or excess added sugar. Replace them with gut-friendly staples like:

- Canned green beans, peas, and carrots
- Canned peaches and pears in 100% juice or light syrup
- Canola or olive oil
- Corn flakes
- Cream of rice
- Cream of wheat
- Creamy nut or seed butters
- Crisped rice cereal
- Flour tortillas
- Garlic- and shallot-infused olive oil (these add flavor without causing discomfort)
- Rice cakes
- Saltine or oyster crackers
- Spices like cinnamon, ginger, and turmeric
- Sweet potatoes
- Unsweetened applesauce
- Vegetable juice
- Waffle and pancake mix
- White bread
- White pasta
- White potatoes
- White rice

Fridge Favorites

You may also need to make some refrigerator swaps to focus more on gentle, whole foods. Rotate stock of these items depending on the meals you are planning each week to maintain a variety of vitamins and minerals in your diet. Stock your refrigerator with these fresh staples:

- 100% fruit juice (no additives)
- Asparagus
- Avocado
- Bananas
- Carrots
- Eggs
- Green beans
- Lactose-free milk (or nondairy alternatives like almond milk or soymilk)
- Lactose-free pudding or ice cream
- Low-fat buttery spread (nondairy)
- Low-fat Greek yogurt (or nondairy alternative)
- Mushrooms
- Peeled apples
- Salmon
- Skinless chicken or turkey
- Squash
- Tofu
- Trout

These lists are all general and inclusive. There is no need for you to stock your pantry or fridge with foods you are sensitive to, such as dairy or wheat. Customize these lists to fit your unique needs.

SOURCES OF OMEGA-3 FATTY ACIDS

There seems to be a lot of hype around omega-3 fatty acids (omega-3s), and the hype is completely legitimate! Omega-3s are healthy fats found in plants and fish. Incorporating them into your diet is a great way to both protect your system and reduce inflammation.

Omega-3s are found in three major categories, which you can mix and match depending on your unique dietary needs.

Fatty fish are the best source of omega-3s and are also low-residue, high-protein options for a Crohn's diet. The fish highest in omega-3s are:

- Anchovies
- Mackerel
- Oysters
- Salmon
- Sardines
- Trout

Nuts and seeds are the best plant-based sources of omega-3s, and while whole nuts and seeds can be problematic with Crohn's disease, you can still get maximum benefit from nut butters, seed butters, and ground or soaked seeds like:

- Chia seeds
- Flaxseeds
- Hemp seeds
- Walnuts

Supplements are another way to get omega-3s in your diet, and your doctor or dietitian may recommend one of the following if dietary sources alone are not meeting your needs:

- Fish liver oil supplements (like cod liver oil)
- Fish oil supplements
- Krill oil supplements

Essential Equipment

The recipes in this book are simple to prepare with easy-to-find ingredients. To make the most out of the recipes, a well-stocked kitchen should include:

- Aluminum foil
- Baking sheet
- Blender
- Cutting board
- Mason jars or freezer-safe containers
- Meat thermometer
- Parchment paper
- Sharp knives
- Slotted spoon
- Slow cooker
- Small and large pan or skillet
- Small and large saucepan
- Stockpot or large, deep pan
- Strainer or colander
- Vegetable peeler

About the Recipes

This cookbook has been carefully crafted to include recipes that will work for any person with Crohn's disease, including recipe modifications depending on your specific sensitivities. Although you can enjoy these recipes at any time, each recipe has been labeled to indicate whether it is particularly helpful during a flare-up or during remission. Other labels that can help you quickly ascertain if a recipe is suitable for you include:

Dairy-Free: These recipes are perfect for anyone who is lactose intolerant or experiencing a flare-up.

Gluten-Free: These recipes do not have any ingredients that contain gluten.

Low Fat: Most of the recipes in this book are low fat, because fatty foods are a trigger for most people with Crohn's.

Low Fiber or Low Residue: These recipes are especially helpful during flare-ups and are very gentle on the system.

Low FODMAP: These recipes may not exclude all FODMAPs, but they will be low FODMAP to be gentler on your body.

Paleo: These recipes limit processed foods and exclude grains, dairy, legumes, and sugar. They are gentle and suitable for most people with Crohn's.

All the ingredients in the recipes have been carefully selected to help you eat a variety of great-tasting foods on a Crohn's diet. With these 100 recipes, you can easily create a weekly or monthly menu and never be bored. Furthermore, each recipe contains helpful tips and variations, such as:

Ingredient Tip: More information about a specific ingredient, such as how to select and purchase it, best practices, and nutrition facts.

Make Ahead: Many recipes can be made ahead and reheated to cut down on cooking time during the week.

Make It Easier: Tips or shortcuts to make the cooking process easier.

Make It Milder: Methods or swaps to make the recipe even milder on your system.

Substitution: Suggested ingredient substitutions to vary the dish or accommodate a dietary restriction or potential trigger.

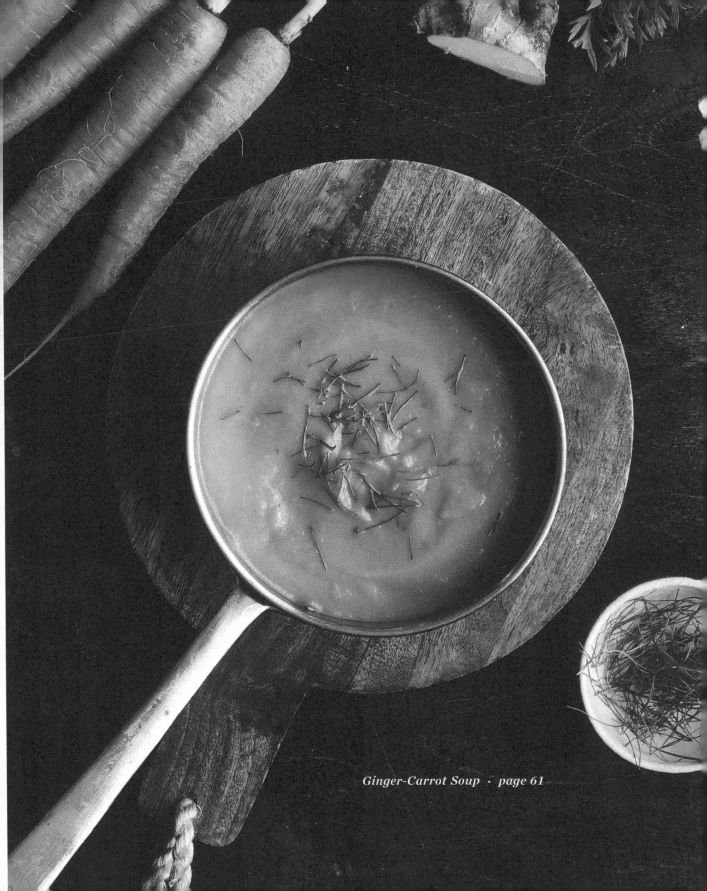

Ginger-Carrot Soup · page 61

CHAPTER 3

Meal Plans

Meal planning is a truly valuable approach to eating specific food groups and is something anyone can do to save time, money, and ensure a variety of nutrients in their diet.

I have prepared two sample meal plans for you in this chapter, one for a flare-up week and another for a week of remission. The purpose of these is to guide you through avoiding foods that trigger or aggravate flares. No one meal plan suits every person with Crohn's, so it is important to modify these based on your individual needs.

The beauty of meal plans is that they take the guesswork out of what to eat. After using a meal plan as a guide for one week, you can build your own for subsequent weeks and fill them with your favorite recipes.

Meal Planning and Prepping

A meal plan, at its simplest, is a list of the things you would like to eat in a day or a week. It gives you control over what food you put into your body, reducing the number of surprise flare-ups that may come from eating without a plan in place.

Meal prepping involves making your whole recipes or parts of recipes ahead of time, such as prepping a large batch of ingredients or meals on a Sunday to eat throughout the week. Having ready-to-eat items available takes the stress out of having to prepare something if you are not feeling well or are in a time crunch.

Use these tips to successfully prep your meals ahead:

- Keep your pantry and refrigerator stocked with staples (see pages 28 and 29) to ensure you always have Crohn's-friendly ingredients on hand.

- Have a small stock of glass food storage containers to preportion your meals. Glass is freezer-safe, microwave-safe, and dishwasher safe. You can buy freezer-safe mason jars for soups, and Pyrex makes very affordable storage containers in a variety of portion-friendly sizes that are sold at most major retailers.

- After you make your meal plan for the week, identify any recipes that can be made ahead of time—such as a slow-cooker soup that can cook while you are at work and be stored once you get home.

- Try doubling the recipe you are already cooking and storing the additional portions for future meals.

Meal Plan for Flare-Ups

When you are experiencing a flare-up, meal planning, grocery shopping, and cooking may be the last things you want to do. A simple way to eliminate stress during a flare-up is to have preplanned meals that are easy to prepare and gentle on your system.

This is a sample meal plan for one week that is fit for a flare-up. These recipes are quick to prepare, require minimal ingredients, and are delicious, low-fiber, and dairy-free, while remaining nutritious and soothing to your system. You can use this meal plan to make a weekly grocery list so that you have food on hand if you start to feel a flare-up coming on. Look ahead into the week. If there is something you have time to prepare in advance, you will have ready-made lunches or dinners available.

Meal Plan for Flare-Ups

	BREAKFAST	LUNCH	DINNER
MON	Cinnamon and Nutmeg-Spiced Oatmeal (page 48)	Chicken Salad Wraps (page 82)	Ginger Shrimp with Sticky Rice (page 131)
TUE	Melon Smoothie (page 44)	Egg Drop Soup (page 58) with "Everything" Tofu (page 100)	Mushroom Pasta (page 158)
WED	Savory Hot Cereal (page 49)	Pasta Salad (page 81)	Honey-Mustard Salmon (page 140)
THUR	Avocado Toast (page 46)	Cream-less Potato Soup (page 62)	Chicken-Vegetable Lasagna (page 118)
FRI	Breakfast Rice (page 50)	Bone Broth (page 72)	Étouffée (page 150)
SAT	Egg Bake (page 54)	Paella (page 152)	Sweet Potato–Quinoa Chicken Salad (page 84)
SUN	Zucchini Bread (page 47)	Tuna Salad (page 87)	Fried Rice (page 144) with Ginger-Carrot Soup (page 61)

A NOTE ON MEAL SIZE

Eating smaller, more frequent meals can ease some of the work your digestive system is doing. Eating too much in one sitting can make it need to work harder or longer, which can increase discomfort and symptoms. Slowing down, chewing your food thoroughly, and listening to your body can help you stop eating before you reach the point of over-fullness.

Preparing meals ahead of time is a great way to preportion your meals in amounts you know you tolerate well. Feel free to modify the amounts and number of times per day you eat to suit your body.

Meal Plan for Remission

Meal planning is useful not only during a flare-up, but also during remission or whenever you are experiencing minimal symptoms. Use this meal plan to maximize the variety of nutrients in your diet when you are feeling better. Remission is a great time to nourish your body to replenish nutrient stores that may get depleted during flare-ups. These recipes have been chosen and placed throughout the week to boost nutrition and add variety. They are still gentle on the digestive system but include more fiber and meat than the recipes chosen for a flare-up. You will find items such as berries, peanut butter, and various vegetables added.

Meal Plan for Remission

	BREAKFAST	LUNCH	DINNER
MON	Berry Smoothie (page 42)	Turkey Lettuce Wraps with Mango and Avocado (page 86)	Pork Tenderloin with Sweet Potatoes (page 123)
TUE	Chicken Omelet (page 53)	Burrito Bowl (page 102)	Tofu Stir-Fry (page 101)
WED	Tropical Smoothie (page 43)	Simple "Sushi" Bowls (page 132)	Pasta with Avocado Pesto (page 153)
THUR	Veggie Scramble (page 52)	Chicken Cobb Salad (page 83)	Vegetable Enchiladas (page 103) with Spanish Rice (page 149)
FRI	Peanut Butter–Banana Smoothie (page 45)	Veggie Pitas (page 95)	Chicken and Eggs (page 111)
SAT	Avocado Toast (page 46)	Fish Tacos (page 137)	Turmeric Chicken and Potatoes (page 114)
SUN	Egg Bake (page 54)	Gumbo (page 67)	Pad Thai (page 104)

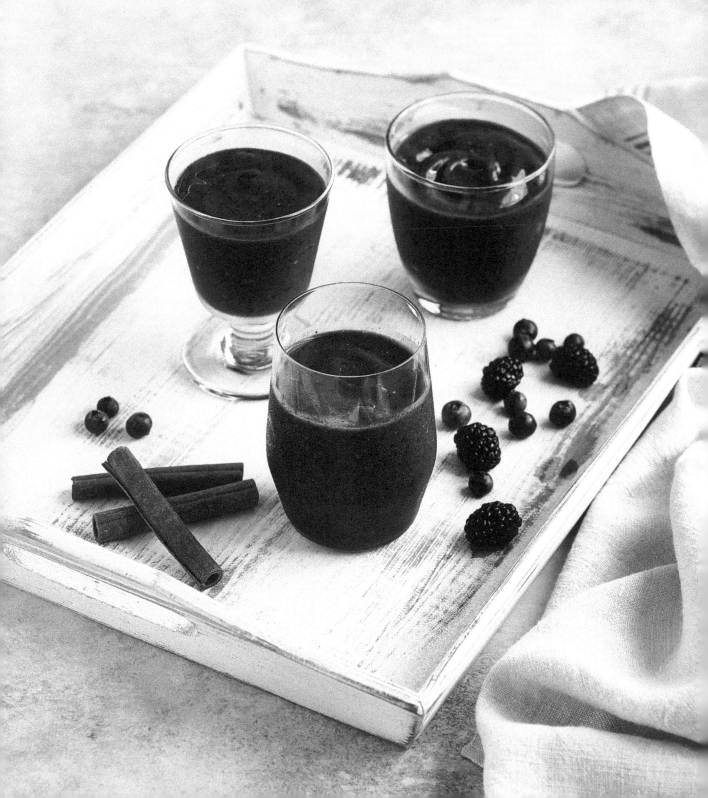

Berry Smoothie · page 42

CHAPTER 4

Smoothies & Breakfasts

Breakfast is often said to be the most important meal of the day. Though it may not be the most important for you, starting your morning with nutrition in your body is a great way to ease your system into the day with energy and sustenance.

Berry Smoothie

PREP TIME 5 MINUTES ✖ **SERVES** 2 TO 4

REMISSION · DAIRY-FREE · GLUTEN-FREE · LOW FAT · PALEO

_____

A cool, refreshing smoothie with a perfect blend of sweet and tart berries, plus a hint of spice from the cinnamon, is a great way to start your day. Berries and cinnamon are both anti-inflammatory superstars, making this smoothie a winner for eating with Crohn's.

1 cup frozen blueberries

1 cup frozen raspberries

1 cup frozen blackberries

1 teaspoon ground cinnamon

2 cups unsweetened plain or vanilla almond milk

1. Place all the ingredients in a blender and blend on high, or on the smoothie setting, for 30 to 60 seconds, until smooth.
2. Add additional liquid as needed and reblend.
3. Serve chilled.

make it milder: To reduce fiber in this recipe during a flare-up, you can substitute 100% berry juice and 3 cups of ice in place of the frozen berries. You will retain the anti-inflammatory benefits of the berries but make it easier to digest the smoothie without the berry skins or seeds.

make ahead: You can make this smoothie ahead of time by portioning it into freezer-safe mason jars and freezing. To thaw, simply put a portion in the refrigerator the night before you want to enjoy it for breakfast. You may want to give the smoothie a good shake before drinking it.

_____

Per Serving: Calories: 108; Total Fat: 2g; Saturated Fat: 0g; Total Carbohydrates: 22g; Fiber: 7g; Sugars: 13g; Protein: 2g

Tropical Smoothie

PREP TIME 5 MINUTES ✖ **SERVES** 2 TO 4

FLARE-UP · REMISSION · DAIRY-FREE · GLUTEN-FREE · LOW FAT · LOW FIBER · LOW FODMAP

Pineapple, papaya, and banana are low-FODMAP fruits that are full of important nutrients, vitamins, and minerals. While pineapple has a bit more fiber, papaya and banana are low-fiber/low-residue fruits. During a flare-up, replace the pineapple with an extra papaya for lower fiber.

1 (14-ounce) can pineapple chunks in 100% juice (no sugar added), juice reserved

1 papaya, skinned, pitted and cubed

2 bananas, peeled and sliced

1 teaspoon ground ginger

1 teaspoon ground turmeric

1 cup ice

1. Combine all the ingredients in a blender and blend on high, or on the smoothie setting, for 30 to 60 seconds.
2. Add additional liquid as needed and reblend.
3. Serve chilled.

make it easier: Any time you have leftover fruit, freeze it to reduce food waste and make prep easy for your next smoothie.

make ahead: You can make this smoothie ahead of time by portioning it into freezer-safe mason jars and freezing. To thaw, simply put a portion in the refrigerator the night before you want to enjoy it for breakfast. You may need to give the smoothie a good shake before drinking it.

Per Serving: Calories: 146; Total Fat: 0g; Saturated Fat: 0g; Total Carbohydrates: 36g; Fiber: 4g; Sugars: 25g; Protein: 2g

Melon Smoothie

PREP TIME 5 MINUTES ✳ **SERVES** 2 TO 4

FLARE-UP · REMISSION · DAIRY-FREE · GLUTEN-FREE · LOW FAT · LOW FIBER

Melons are a wonderful fruit for any diet, but especially when eating for Crohn's, because of their low fiber and low residue levels. Deliciously crisp without being overly sweet, this melon smoothie will start your day on a bright note.

2 cucumbers, peeled, seeded, and cut into chunks

½ cantaloupe, seeded and cut into chunks

½ honeydew melon, seeded and cut into chunks

1 tablespoon lime juice

2 cups ice

1. Put all the ingredients into a blender and blend on high, or on the smoothie setting, for 30 to 60 seconds.
2. Serve chilled.

make it easier: Any time you have leftover cucumber or melon, pop it into a freezer-safe bag or container, and you'll have smoothie-ready ingredients for next time.

make ahead: You can make this smoothie ahead of time by portioning it into freezer-safe mason jars and freezing. To thaw, simply put a portion in the refrigerator the night before you want to enjoy it for breakfast. You may need to give the smoothie a good shake before drinking it.

Per Serving: Calories: 98; Total Fat: 1g; Saturated Fat: 0g; Total Carbohydrates: 24g; Fiber: 3g; Sugars: 20g; Protein: 2g

Peanut Butter–Banana Smoothie

PREP TIME 5 MINUTES ⁂ **SERVES** 2 TO 4

REMISSION · DAIRY-FREE · GLUTEN-FREE · LOW FODMAP

Because peanuts are a low-FODMAP nut, creamy natural peanut butter made entirely from peanuts is a great Crohn's-friendly food. Peanut butter and banana is a comforting, nostalgic flavor combination, and together they provide a dose of protein and easy-to-digest carbohydrates.

4 cups frozen sliced bananas

½ cup natural creamy peanut butter

2 cups unsweetened plain or vanilla almond milk

1. Combine all the ingredients in a blender and blend on high, or on the smoothie setting, for 30 to 60 seconds.
2. Add additional liquid and reblend for a looser smoothie, or add a few ice cubes and reblend for a thicker smoothie.
3. Serve chilled.

ingredient tip: Freezing bananas before they go bad is a perfect way to have frozen bananas ready for smoothies. Simply slice the overripe bananas and freeze in a freezer-safe container or bag.

Per Serving: Calories: 462; Total Fat: 24g; Saturated Fat: 4g; Total Carbohydrates: 56g; Fiber: 8g; Sugars: 30g; Protein: 14g

Avocado Toast

Avocados are a Crohn's superfood because they are packed with nutrients, easy on your digestive system, and delicious! Avocados are high in B vitamins, and the healthy fats they contain help your body absorb fat-soluble vitamins.

1 large avocado

2 to 4 slices of white bread

2 tablespoons olive oil

2 teaspoons lemon juice

Salt

1. Slice the avocado and divide it into 2 to 4 portions, depending on how many slices of avocado toast you are preparing. Set aside.
2. Toast the bread to your liking.
3. Top the toast with the avocado slices.
4. Drizzle the avocado toast with olive oil and lemon juice. Sprinkle with salt and serve.

substitution: Feel free to use gluten-free bread if gluten or wheat are triggers for you. Any bread you like and that makes you feel good works perfectly in this preparation.

ingredient tip: An avocado is ripe when the skin is purple to black, with little to no green, and it yields to gentle pressure. If it feels firm, it is not ripe yet, and if it feels mushy, it is overly ripe.

Per Serving: Calories: 160; Total Fat: 12g; Saturated Fat: 2g; Total Carbohydrates: 11g; Fiber: 4g; Sugars: 1g; Protein: 3g

Zucchini Bread

PREP TIME 15 MINUTES ⁂ **COOK TIME** 1 HOUR, PLUS 10 MINUTES TO COOL ⁂ **SERVES** 6 TO 8

FLARE-UP · REMISSION · DAIRY-FREE · LOW FAT · LOW FIBER

When fall comes around, I start craving zucchini bread and always eat more than my fair share of it! No matter the season, zucchini is a delicious, inexpensive vegetable that is easy to digest.

1 medium or large zucchini, peeled and seeded

¼ cup canola or vegetable oil

1 cup unsweetened applesauce

2 teaspoons vanilla extract

1½ cups all-purpose flour

½ cup sugar

1 teaspoon baking soda

1 teaspoon ground cinnamon

1 teaspoon ground ginger

½ teaspoon baking powder

½ teaspoon ground nutmeg

1. Preheat the oven to 350°F. Line a 9-by-5-inch loaf pan with parchment paper.

2. Grate the zucchini into a large bowl. Add the oil, applesauce, and vanilla, and mix until the zucchini is well coated in the wet ingredients.

3. In another large bowl, whisk together the flour, sugar, baking soda, cinnamon, ginger, baking powder, and nutmeg.

4. Add the wet ingredients to the dry ingredients and mix until combined.

5. Pour the mixture into the prepared loaf pan and bake for 50 to 60 minutes, keeping an eye on the bread during the last 10 minutes to prevent burning. The bread is done when a toothpick inserted in the center comes out clean.

6. Allow the bread to cool in the pan for 10 minutes before serving.

substitution: You can easily make this recipe gluten-free by swapping the flour for your favorite gluten-free flour. Many gluten-free flours can replace flour 1-to-1, but some might require a gluten substitute like xanthan gum. The ratio is 1 teaspoon of gluten substitute per 1 cup of gluten-free flour.

make ahead: You can double or triple this batch and make several loaves to store in your freezer for up to 3 months. Simply thaw in the refrigerator overnight before serving.

Per Serving: Calories: 210; Total Fat: 7g; Saturated Fat: 1g; Total Carbohydrates: 33g; Fiber: 3g; Sugars: 16g; Protein: 3g

Cinnamon and Nutmeg–Spiced Oatmeal

PREP TIME 5 MINUTES ✳ **COOK TIME** 5 MINUTES ✳ **SERVES** 2

FLARE-UP · REMISSION · DAIRY-FREE · GLUTEN-FREE · LOW FAT

There is something so comforting about a bowl of oatmeal. It takes us back to simpler times in our lives, and it makes us feel like we are making a healthy choice for the body. Many oatmeal packets are loaded with sugar and ingredients we cannot pronounce, so making this spiced oatmeal at home is a true win.

1 cup water

½ cup rolled oats

1 teaspoon honey

1 teaspoon ground cinnamon

½ teaspoon ground nutmeg

1. In a small bowl, combine the water, oats, honey, cinnamon, and nutmeg.
2. Microwave on high for 2 minutes.
3. Stir and allow the oatmeal to sit for 2 minutes.
4. Serve warm.

ingredient tip: Oatmeal is a great Crohn's staple, but certain types of oats are better for your gut than others. Steel-cut oats are generally popular because of their high fiber content, but for you, rolled oats may be a better choice. You get the benefits of oats without the high residue.

make ahead: For an even easier preparation, make this recipe "overnight" style. Before bed, simply combine all the ingredients—using 1 cup of oats instead of ½ cup—in a mason jar or airtight container. Leave the oats in the refrigerator overnight, and breakfast will be ready and waiting for you morning!

Per Serving: Calories: 93; Total Fat: 2g; Saturated Fat: 0g; Total Carbohydrates: 18g; Fiber: 3g; Sugars: 3g; Protein: 3g

Savory Hot Cereal

PREP TIME 5 MINUTES ✳ **COOK TIME** 10 MINUTES ✳ **SERVES** 2

FLARE-UP · REMISSION · DAIRY-FREE · LOW FAT

Traditionally, Cream of Wheat is prepared with butter, milk, and sugar. This version is far more digestion friendly, with an extra boost of protein and a fresh, savory flavor instead of the typical sweet version.

2 cups water

⅓ cup Cream of Wheat

1 teaspoon fresh or dried dill

Salt

2 teaspoons canola oil

2 eggs

1. In a medium saucepan, bring the water to a boil.
2. When the water in the saucepan reaches a boil, add the Cream of Wheat, dill, and a sprinkle of salt, whisking constantly until it is well incorporated in the water.
3. Cook the cereal for 2 to 3 minutes, until it thickens.
4. Meanwhile, in a small pan or skillet, heat the oil over medium-high heat until shimmering.
5. Crack the eggs into the skillet, cover with a lid, and cook for 3 to 8 minutes, depending on how you like your eggs. (For a sunny-side-up egg, remove from the pan after 3 minutes of cooking. For an over-easy egg, flip and cook for 1 more minute. For an over-medium egg, cook for 3 more minutes. For an over-hard egg, cook for 5 more minutes.)
6. Serve each bowl of cereal with an egg on top and a sprinkle of salt.

make it milder: During a flare-up, you can omit the egg in this recipe to make it even gentler on your system.

substitution: The mild flavor of the Cream of Wheat will go well with anything you feel like adding, like spinach or avocado. Feel free to add whatever works well for your body.

Per Serving: Calories: 132; Total Fat: 9g; Saturated Fat: 2g; Total Carbohydrates: 5g; Fiber: 0g; Sugars: 1g; Protein: 6g

Breakfast Rice

PREP TIME 30 MINUTES ❊ COOK TIME 1 HOUR ❊ SERVES 2 TO 4

FLARE-UP · REMISSION · DAIRY-FREE · GLUTEN-FREE · LOW FAT · LOW FIBER · LOW FODMAP

Although rice may not be a common breakfast food in America, it is often eaten for breakfast in many other parts of the world. Sometimes called congee, breakfast rice has a porridge-like texture with a creamy (but dairy-free) mouthfeel that is comforting and luscious. Think of this breakfast rice like you would oatmeal or cream of wheat.

¾ cup long-grain white rice

2 teaspoons ground ginger

1 teaspoon olive oil

9 cups vegetable stock

1. In a colander, rinse the rice several times.
2. Place the colander in a large stockpot and fill the pot with water to cover the rice. Soak the rice for 30 minutes.
3. Lift the colander out of the pot and discard the water from the pot.
4. In a medium bowl, combine the rice, ginger, and olive oil, coating the rice with the oil.
5. In the same large pot you used for soaking the rice, bring the vegetable stock to a boil.
6. Carefully add the rice to the stock and bring it back to a boil.
7. Reduce the heat to medium and stir the rice for 2 minutes.
8. Reduce the heat to low and set a lid over the pot, leaving a slight gap to let steam escape.

9. Simmer the rice for 45 minutes or until it has a creamy, porridge-like texture.

10. Serve for a nutritious breakfast.

substitution: Feel free to flavor this recipe with any spices or toppings that are gentle on your system, such as spinach, avocado, egg, soy sauce, or leeks. Rice is a perfect blank canvas to accept other flavors.

make ahead: This breakfast rice requires more time to prepare than your average breakfast. You could make it the night before while you make dinner, since it only requires one extra pot on the stove. You can also make it in a larger batch and portion it out for the week.

Per Serving: Calories: 155; Total Fat: 1g; Saturated Fat: 0g; Total Carbohydrates: 32g; Fiber: 1g; Sugars: 5g; Protein: 2g

Veggie Scramble

PREP TIME 5 MINUTES ✳ **COOK TIME** 10 MINUTES ✳ **SERVES** 2 TO 4

REMISSION · DAIRY-FREE · GLUTEN-FREE · LOW FODMAP · PALEO

———————————

Scrambled eggs are a quick, simple, protein-rich breakfast that is easy on the gut. Making the perfect scrambled eggs is simple and takes only a few minutes. This recipe includes vegetables that are easy to digest.

1 tablespoon canola oil

4 eggs

½ cup unsweetened plain nondairy milk

½ red bell pepper, skin and seeds removed, diced

½ cup chopped spinach

2 tablespoons dried chives or minced fresh chives

1 teaspoon dried oregano

Salt

1. In a large pan or skillet, heat the oil over medium heat until shimmering.
2. In a large bowl, whisk the eggs and nondairy milk together until well mixed.
3. Add the bell pepper, spinach, chives, oregano, and a sprinkle of salt, and stir until all ingredients are well combined.
4. Pour the egg mixture into the pan.
5. Using a spatula, as the egg cooks, slowly move it from the edges of the pan to the center. The liquid mixture will flow to the edges to cook. Repeat until the eggs are cooked to your desired consistency, about 8 minutes.
6. Serve warm.

make it milder: To make this recipe milder, you can cook the vegetables for 3 to 5 minutes first, then add the whisked eggs to the pan. The longer you cook the vegetables, short of burning them, the easier they will be to digest.

substitution: If you can tolerate cheese, adding it would add protein and calcium to this delicious scramble.

———————————

Per Serving: Calories: 109; Total Fat: 9g; Saturated Fat: 2g; Total Carbohydrates: 2g; Fiber: 1g; Sugars: 1g; Protein: 6g

Chicken Omelet

PREP TIME 5 MINUTES ※ COOK TIME 10 MINUTES ※ SERVES 2 TO 4

REMISSION · DAIRY-FREE · GLUTEN-FREE · LOW FIBER · LOW FODMAP · PALEO

Vegetables are certainly welcome in this savory omelet, made fresh with Crohn's-friendly diced tomatoes, which are conveniently skinless and seedless when canned, plus nutrient-rich spinach and olives. Chicken may not be what comes to mind for breakfast, but it is a great way to use leftovers—not to mention that the mild flavor blends in perfectly with the eggs and adds a protein boost to the start of your day.

1 tablespoon olive oil

6 eggs

1 cup canned diced tomatoes, drained

1 (2.25-ounce) can sliced black olives

1 cup chopped spinach, fresh or frozen

½ cup cooked shredded or diced chicken

Salt

1. In a large pan or skillet, heat the oil over medium heat until shimmering.
2. In the meantime, in a large bowl, whisk the eggs until the whites and yolks are well mixed.
3. Add the diced tomatoes, olives, spinach, and chicken to the eggs. Stir until everything is evenly distributed.
4. Pour the egg mixture into the pan and cook for 5 minutes or until the edges begin to loosen from the pan and the egg on the surface begins to set.
5. Flip the omelet over and cook for an additional 5 minutes.
6. Serve with a sprinkle of salt.

make it milder: If meat is not friendly to your system, feel free to omit the chicken in this recipe. If chicken sits well with you, the small amount here adds an extra bit of protein and texture.

substitution: If cheese is gentle for you, adding cheese to this recipe would add some protein and calcium, as well as a luscious texture.

Per Serving: Calories: 215; Total Fat: 14g; Saturated Fat: 3g; Total Carbohydrates: 4g; Fiber: 2g; Sugars: 2g; Protein: 19g

Egg Bake

PREP TIME 5 MINUTES ❋ **COOK TIME** 1 HOUR, PLUS 5 MINUTES TO COOL ❋ **SERVES** 6 TO 8

FLARE-UP · REMISSION · DAIRY-FREE · GLUTEN-FREE · LOW FIBER · LOW FODMAP · PALEO

This casserole-style breakfast can easily feed a crowd or last you for several meals. Since it is filled with hearty eggs and potatoes, you could also eat this for lunch or dinner. Eggs aren't just for breakfast, after all.

Nonstick cooking spray, for greasing the baking dish
1 dozen eggs
1 cup unsweetened plain nondairy milk

1 zucchini, peeled, seeded, and chopped
2 cups fresh spinach, chopped
1 (30-ounce) package hash browns

1 tablespoon dried basil
2 teaspoons dried or rubbed sage
1 teaspoon ground thyme
Salt

1. Preheat the oven to 350°F. Coat a 9-by-13-inch baking dish with nonstick cooking spray.

2. In a large bowl, whisk together the eggs and nondairy milk until well mixed.

3. Add the zucchini, spinach, hash browns, basil, sage, thyme, and a sprinkle of salt to the eggs. Stir together until all ingredients are evenly distributed.

4. Pour the egg mixture into the prepared baking dish.

5. Bake uncovered for 1 hour. During the last 15 minutes, watch to make sure the edges are not burning.

6. Allow the egg bake to cool for 5 minutes, then serve.

ingredient tip: Frozen or fresh hash browns work equally well in this preparation, because it is all baked in the oven together. Using frozen hash browns can save both time and money, since you can buy large bags of them.

make ahead: This is a perfect make-ahead breakfast, because it can be portioned out for the week and refrigerated for up to 1 week or frozen for up to 2 months.

Per Serving: Calories: 388; Total Fat: 21g; Saturated Fat: 6g; Total Carbohydrates: 38g; Fiber: 4g; Sugars: 3g; Protein: 12g

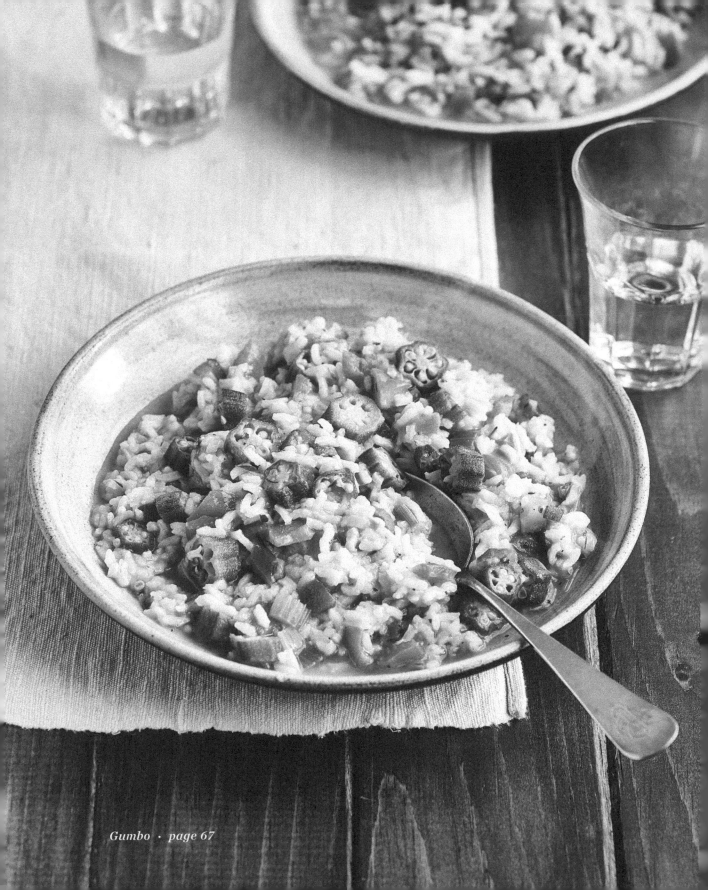

Gumbo · page 67

CHAPTER 5

Soups

Soup provides warmth, comfort, and nutrition in a time-saving fashion. The secret is that the best soups do not come out of a can... they come out of your kitchen.

Egg Drop Soup

PREP TIME 5 MINUTES ✳ **COOK TIME** 10 MINUTES ✳ **SERVES** 2 TO 4

FLARE-UP · REMISSION · DAIRY-FREE · LOW FIBER · LOW FODMAP · PALEO

———————————

Egg drop soup is a staple at Chinese restaurants that is sometimes more delicious than the main dish. The secret is that you can make your own at home and it will be just as good!

3 eggs

1 tablespoon cornstarch

1 tablespoon cold water

1 (32-ounce) container chicken stock

¼ teaspoon ground ginger

Sesame oil (optional)

Soy sauce

1. In a medium bowl, whisk the eggs.

2. In a small bowl, whisk together the cornstarch and cold water to make a slurry.

3. In a large stockpot over medium heat, bring the chicken stock and ginger to a simmer.

4. Add the cornstarch slurry to the broth, stirring constantly for 10 seconds.

5. Continue stirring while you pour in the beaten eggs in a thin, steady stream. Stir constantly to evenly cook the egg in wispy ribbons.

6. Serve each bowl with a drizzle of sesame oil, if desired, and soy sauce to taste.

ingredient tip: Egg drop soup does not reheat well, but that's okay, because it is so quick to prepare. You can have a fresh bowl in under 15 minutes.

———————————

Per Serving: Calories: 141; Total Fat: 6g; Saturated Fat: 2g; Total Carbohydrates: 10g; Fiber: 0g; Sugars: 4g; Protein: 10g

Avocado-Pea Soup

PREP TIME 15 MINUTES ❈ **COOK TIME** 20 MINUTES ❈ **SERVES** 2 TO 4

FLARE-UP · REMISSION · DAIRY-FREE · GLUTEN-FREE · LOW FAT · PALEO

This vibrant green soup includes healthy fats from avocado, plus protein and carbohydrates from peas and anti-inflammatory nutrients from both. It's a tasty, nutrient-filled choice that's easy on the body.

2 avocados

2 tablespoons olive oil

1 bunch fresh parsley

2 cups vegetable stock

3 cups frozen peas

½ teaspoon salt

1. Slice the avocados in half, remove the pits, and scoop the flesh from the skins.

2. Put the avocado flesh, oil, and parsley in a blender and blend on high, or on the smoothie setting, for 30 to 60 seconds. Leave the mixture in the blender and set it aside.

3. In a large stockpot over medium heat, combine the vegetable stock, peas, and salt.

4. Cover the pot and simmer for 20 minutes.

5. Remove the pot from the heat, add the avocado mixture, and stir to combine.

6. Transfer the soup to a blender in four small batches. For each batch, cover tightly and puree on high, or on the smoothie setting, for 30 to 60 seconds. Transfer the pureed soup to a serving bowl.

7. Serve warm or chilled.

make it milder: The longer you have to let the peas cook and break down, the easier they are to digest. Peas are generally gentle on the system, despite being legumes.

ingredient tip: Canned peas work just as well in this preparation, but they will have a less bright flavor. They are nutritionally equivalent to fresh or frozen peas, but higher in sodium. Simply drain and rinse the canned peas to remove most of the excess sodium.

Per Serving: Calories: 258; Total Fat: 18g; Saturated Fat: 3g; Total Carbohydrates: 21g; Fiber: 10g; Sugars: 6g; Protein: 7g

Asparagus-Potato Soup

PREP TIME 10 MINUTES ✕ **COOK TIME** 35 MINUTES ✕ **SERVES** 4

FLARE-UP · REMISSION · DAIRY-FREE · GLUTEN-FREE · LOW FAT · LOW FIBER · PALEO

This is a great recipe for a fridge clean-out, since you can add any vegetables that are leftover or past their prime. Feel free to make this soup with your favorite Crohn's-friendly vegetables.

1 bunch asparagus

4 medium potatoes, peeled

3 carrots, peeled

1 tablespoon olive oil

1 (32-ounce) container vegetable stock

2 tablespoons dried parsley

1 cup unsweetened plain nondairy milk

1. Trim and discard the woody ends of the asparagus. Then, roughly chop the asparagus, potatoes, and carrots.

2. In a large stockpot over medium heat, heat the oil until shimmering.

3. Add the chopped vegetables and cook for 10 minutes or until fork-tender.

4. Pour in the stock and add the parsley. Cover and simmer for 25 minutes.

5. Carefully transfer the soup to a blender in four small batches. For each batch, add ¼ cup nondairy milk, cover tightly, and puree on high, or on the smoothie setting, for 30 to 60 seconds. Transfer the pureed soup to a serving bowl.

6. Serve with soft bread.

make ahead: This soup freezes beautifully. Simply portion it into freezer-safe bags or containers and freeze it for up to 6 months. To thaw, leave a bag in the refrigerator overnight, and microwave the soup or heat it on the stove when you are ready to eat.

Per Serving: Calories: 258; Total Fat: 5g; Saturated Fat: 1g; Total Carbohydrates: 49g; Fiber: 8g; Sugars: 9g; Protein: 8g

Ginger-Carrot Soup

PREP TIME 5 MINUTES ✳ **COOK TIME** 20 MINUTES ✳ **SERVES** 4

FLARE-UP · REMISSION · DAIRY-FREE · GLUTEN-FREE · LOW FAT · LOW FIBER · LOW FODMAP

Simple dishes are often the most delicious. This soup allows the flavor of the carrots to shine and gets an added anti-inflammatory flavor boost from the ginger.

2 tablespoons olive oil
2 pounds carrots, peeled and chopped

1 (32-ounce) container chicken stock
2 teaspoons ground ginger

1 cup unsweetened plain nondairy milk
1 tablespoon fennel seeds or dried mint, for garnish

1. In a large stockpot over medium-high heat, heat the oil until shimmering.

2. Cook the carrots for 5 minutes, until they are just about to begin caramelizing.

3. Add the chicken stock and ginger and bring the soup to a low boil.

4. Boil the soup for 10 minutes, until the carrots are tender.

5. Remove the soup from the heat, add the nondairy milk, and stir.

6. Transfer the soup to a blender in four small batches. For each batch, cover tightly and puree on high, or on the smoothie setting, for 30 to 60 seconds. Transfer the pureed soup to a serving bowl.

7. Serve each bowl of soup with a garnish of fennel seeds or mint.

substitution: This recipe can be made vegan by using vegetable stock instead of chicken stock. For a creamier texture, you can use 1 cup of coconut cream or silken tofu in place of the nondairy milk. Using silken tofu would also add protein to this soup.

Per Serving: Calories: 184; Total Fat: 8g; Saturated Fat: 1g; Total Carbohydrates: 24g; Fiber: 7g; Sugars: 11g; Protein: 5g

Cream-less Potato Soup

PREP TIME 10 **MINUTES** ※ **COOK TIME** 40 **MINUTES** ※ **SERVES** 4

FLARE-UP · REMISSION · DIARY-FREE · GLUTEN-FREE · LOW FAT · LOW FIBER · LOW FODMAP

This soup is reminiscent of a loaded baked potato, but without the troublesome cheese and sour cream. With a rich and luscious texture, this soup tastes divine and is heartier than a broth-based soup.

4 potatoes, peeled and chopped
1 (32-ounce) container chicken stock
2 bay leaves
1 cup unsweetened plain nondairy milk
1 tablespoon chopped fresh or dried parsley, for garnish

1. In a large stockpot over medium-high heat, bring the potatoes, chicken stock, and bay leaves to a low boil.
2. Boil the soup for 30 minutes or until the potatoes are tender.
3. Remove the bay leaves and discard.
4. Remove the soup from the heat, add the nondairy milk, and stir.
5. Transfer the soup to a blender in four small batches. For each batch, cover tightly and puree on high, or on the smoothie setting, for 30 to 60 seconds. Transfer the pureed soup to a serving bowl.
6. Serve each bowl of soup garnished with parsley.

substitution: This recipe can be made vegan by using vegetable stock instead of chicken stock. For a creamier texture, you can use 1 cup of coconut cream or silken tofu in place of the nondairy milk. Silken tofu would also add protein to this soup.

Per Serving: Calories: 184; Total Fat: 1g; Saturated Fat: 0g; Total Carbohydrates: 39g; Fiber: 5g; Sugars: 2g; Protein: 5g

Roasted Tomato Soup

PREP TIME 10 MINUTES ⁒ **COOK TIME** 35 MINUTES, PLUS 15 MINUTES TO COOL
SERVES 2 TO 4

REMISSION · DAIRY-FREE · GLUTEN-FREE · LOW FAT · LOW FIBER · PALEO

───────────────

This simple tomato soup has a creamy mouthfeel without any dairy. Tomatoes are full of beneficial nutrients that are also gentle on your gut. Removing the skins and seeds from the tomatoes makes this soup low fiber and even easier to digest.

6 pounds beefsteak
  tomatoes
4 tablespoons olive
  oil, divided

¼ teaspoon salt
1 (32-ounce) container
  vegetable stock

¼ cup fresh parsley, minced

1. Preheat the oven to 400°F. Line a baking sheet with parchment paper.
2. While the oven is preheating, halve each tomato and scoop out the seeds with a spoon or melon baller.
3. On the prepared baking sheet, spread the tomato halves in a single layer, cut-side up.
4. Drizzle the tomatoes with 2 tablespoons of olive oil and sprinkle with the salt.
5. Roast the tomatoes in the preheated oven for 20 minutes, turning them over after 10 minutes to prevent burning.
6. Remove the tomatoes from the oven and allow them to cool for 15 minutes.
7. Remove the skins. Running them under cold water will make this easier.

continued...

Roasted Tomato Soup *continued*

8. In a large microwave-safe container, heat the vegetable stock for 3 to 5 minutes.
9. Put the peeled tomatoes, vegetable stock, and parsley in a blender and blend them on high for 30 to 60 seconds.
10. Serve each bowl of soup with a drizzle of the remaining olive oil.

ingredient tip: This recipe calls for beefsteak tomatoes, but you can use any variety. Beefsteak tomatoes are simply large, meaning they take less time to peel than smaller ones.

make it easier: You can use 2 (15-ounce) cans of stewed tomatoes instead of roasting fresh tomatoes. The flavor will still be delicious but slightly less bright.

Per Serving: Calories: 179; Total Fat: 14g; Saturated Fat: 2g; Total Carbohydrates: 13g; Fiber: 3g; Sugars: 9g; Protein: 3g

Pasta e Fagioli

PREP TIME 10 MINUTES ❋ COOK TIME 40 MINUTES ❋ SERVES 4

REMISSION · DAIRY-FREE · LOW FAT

Pasta e fagioli, also called pasta fagioli, is an Italian soup whose name literally means "pasta and beans." While beans can be gas producing, rinsing the beans in this preparation reduces the gas-causing agents, and cooking them until they are very soft makes them easier to digest.

1 (32-ounce) container beef or chicken stock

1 (16-ounce) box small pasta, such as ditalini or shells

1 (16-ounce) can diced tomatoes, drained

1 (16-ounce) can cannellini or great northern beans, drained and well rinsed

2 celery stalks, chopped

2 carrots, peeled and cut into ½-inch dice

2 tablespoons tomato paste

½ tablespoon dried oregano

½ tablespoon dried basil

1 teaspoon ground thyme

Garlic-infused olive oil, for serving

1. In a large stockpot over medium-high heat, combine all the ingredients except the garlic-infused olive oil.

2. Bring the soup to a simmer.

3. Cook uncovered for 30 to 40 minutes, until the beans and vegetables are tender.

4. Serve each bowl with a drizzle of garlic-infused olive oil.

substitution: If beans are rough on your system, use extra pasta or cubed tofu instead.

make it easier: This soup is a great catchall for any of your favorite leftover vegetables from the week.

Per Serving: Calories: 380; Total Fat: 3g; Saturated Fat: 1g; Total Carbohydrates: 74g; Fiber: 15g; Sugars: 7g; Protein: 20g

Minestrone Soup

PREP TIME 10 MINUTES ⁘ **COOK TIME** 40 MINUTES ⁘ **SERVES** 4

FLARE-UP · REMISSION · DAIRY-FREE · LOW FAT · LOW FIBER · LOW FODMAP

Minestrone is a classic Italian soup made from a wide variety of vegetables and grains. The word itself means "thick vegetable soup," and this Crohn's-friendly recipe for it does not disappoint!

1 (32-ounce) container beef or chicken stock

1 (28-ounce) can diced tomatoes, drained

1 (16-ounce) box small pasta, such as ditalini or shells

2 cups water

2 celery stalks, chopped

2 zucchini, peeled, seeded, and chopped

2 tablespoons tomato paste

1 tablespoon dried oregano

½ tablespoon dried basil

Olive oil, for serving

1. In a large stockpot over medium-high heat, combine all the ingredients except the olive oil.

2. Bring the soup to a simmer.

3. Cook uncovered for 30 to 40 minutes, until all the vegetables are tender.

4. Serve each bowl with a drizzle of olive oil.

substitution: If beans sit well with your system, they make a great protein addition to this soup. Cubed tofu would also work well and would absorb the savory flavors. You can add 1 cup of either in step 1.

make it easier: This soup is a great catchall for any of your favorite leftover vegetables from the week. You can easily substitute whatever vegetables you have on hand for the zucchini or celery.

Per Serving: Calories: 239; Total Fat: 3g; Saturated Fat: 1g; Total Carbohydrates: 48g; Fiber: 10g; Sugars: 10g; Protein: 10g

Gumbo

PREP TIME 10 MINUTES ✖ **COOK TIME** 1 HOUR ✖ **SERVES** 4

REMISSION · DAIRY-FREE · GLUTEN-FREE · LOW FAT

Gumbo is a classic Creole dish that typically features shellfish, poultry, or sausage. This meatless preparation does not skimp on the traditional flavors.

1 green bell pepper
3 celery stalks
10 okra pods
2 tablespoons olive oil

½ cup chopped scallions, green parts only, or minced fresh chives
1 cup white rice

2 bay leaves
1 tablespoon dried oregano
1 teaspoon ground thyme
1 (32-ounce) container vegetable stock

1. Cut the bell pepper in half. Scoop out the seeds and white ribs and discard them.

2. Using a vegetable peeler, carefully remove the skin from the bell pepper.

3. Prepare the vegetables by finely chopping the bell pepper and celery and slicing the okra into ½-inch-thick rounds.

4. In a large stockpot over medium heat, heat the olive oil until shimmering.

5. Cook the bell pepper, celery, okra, and scallions over medium heat for 5 to 10 minutes, until they begin to soften.

6. Add the rice, bay leaves, oregano, thyme, and vegetable stock. Cover, increase the heat to medium high, and cook for 45 minutes.

7. Remove the bay leaves and discard.

8. Serve with soft white bread.

substitution: If beans or tofu sit well with your system, 1 to 2 cups of either, added in step 5, would provide a great protein boost to this gumbo.

ingredient tip: You can serve the gumbo as soon as the rice is tender, but stewing the ingredients together for longer really allows the flavors to marry.

Per Serving: Calories: 147; Total Fat: 8g; Saturated Fat: 1g; Total Carbohydrates: 18g; Fiber: 3g; Sugars: 2g; Protein: 2g

Vegetable Stew

PREP TIME 15 MINUTES ✻ **COOK TIME 40 MINUTES** ✻ **SERVES 4**

FLARE-UP · REMISSION · DAIRY-FREE · GLUTEN-FREE · LOW FAT · LOW FIBER · LOW FODMAP

Vegetable stew is a comforting, safe meal that is gentle on the system. This recipe in particular is low fiber and low FODMAP, making it even gentler than other variations.

2 potatoes, peeled and cut into ½-inch dice

1 sweet potato, peeled and cut into ½-inch dice

2 carrots, peeled and chopped

2 celery stalks, chopped

1 cup chopped fresh spinach

1 (16-ounce) can green beans, drained

1 (16-ounce) can diced tomatoes, drained

1 tablespoon tomato paste

1 (32-ounce) container beef stock

2 cups water

1. In a large stockpot over medium-high heat, combine all the ingredients.
2. Bring the soup to a simmer.
3. Cook uncovered for 30 to 40 minutes, until all the vegetables are tender.
4. Serve with soft bread.

substitution: Vary this recipe with any of your favorite vegetables for different flavors. You can also add meat if your system tolerates it.

make ahead: You can make this recipe in a slow cooker. Put all the ingredients in the slow cooker and cook them on low for at least 6 hours.

Per Serving: Calories: 198; Total Fat: 1g; Saturated Fat: 0g; Total Carbohydrates: 43g; Fiber: 10g; Sugars: 12g; Protein: 9g

Chicken-Leek Soup

PREP TIME 15 MINUTES ✖ **COOK TIME** 45 MINUTES ✖ **SERVES** 4

REMISSION · DAIRY-FREE · GLUTEN-FREE · LOW FIBER · LOW FODMAP

Imagine coming home after a long day to a bowl of chicken soup with a fragrant broth and tender vegetables. The scent alone will calm your senses and excite your palate.

2 tablespoons canola oil

½ pound boneless, skinless chicken breast, cut into 1-inch chunks

2 leeks, thinly sliced

1 zucchini, peeled and seeded

2 potatoes, peeled and cut into ½-inch dice

1 (32-ounce) container chicken stock

4 cups water

1 tablespoon ground turmeric

1. In a large stockpot over medium heat, heat the oil until shimmering.
2. Cook the chicken for 5 minutes, stirring occasionally, until no pink is visible on the outside of each piece.
3. Add the leeks and cook for 5 more minutes.
4. Add the zucchini, potatoes, chicken stock, water, and turmeric, and stir.
5. Allow the soup to simmer for at least 30 minutes, until the potatoes are tender.
6. Serve warm.

substitution: This recipe includes a small amount of chicken. If meat is hard on your system, feel free to omit the chicken in this recipe. If the chicken sits easy with your system, feel free to double the amount of chicken.

make it easier: To save time, you can use leftover cooked chicken in this recipe. Simply skip step 2 and add the chicken with the leeks in step 3.

Per Serving: Calories: 330; Total Fat: 11g; Saturated Fat: 2g; Total Carbohydrates: 29g; Fiber: 4g; Sugars: 4g; Protein: 29g

Chicken and Rice Soup

PREP TIME 10 MINUTES ❈ **COOK TIME** 30 MINUTES ❈ **SERVES** 4

FLARE-UP · REMISSION · DAIRY-FREE · GLUTEN-FREE · LOW FIBER · LOW FODMAP

Chicken soup is a comforting classic. Whether it's made with noodles or rice—or even tiny pasta stars—there is something instantly soothing and restorative about a bowl of chicken soup. Even better, it is nutritious and easy to digest.

2 cups chopped or shredded cooked chicken

3 carrots, cut into ½-inch dice

2 celery stalks, cut into ½-inch dice

1 cup white rice

1 (32-ounce) container chicken stock

4 cups water

1 tablespoon dried parsley

1. In a large stockpot over medium-high heat, combine the chicken, carrots, celery, rice, stock, water, and parsley.

2. Bring the soup to a boil.

3. Reduce the heat to medium low and simmer for 25 minutes or until the rice is tender.

4. Serve warm.

substitution: If chicken does not sit well with your gut during a flare-up, replace the chicken and chicken stock in this recipe with Bone Broth (page 72).

make ahead: This soup can be portioned and stored in airtight containers in the refrigerator for up to 4 days.

Per Serving (1 cup): Calories: 136; Total Fat: 2g; Saturated Fat: 0g; Total Carbohydrates: 17g; Fiber: 2g; Sugars: 3g; Protein: 12g

Pho

PREP TIME 10 MINUTES ⁂ COOK TIME 45 MINUTES ⁂ SERVES 4

FLARE-UP · REMISSION · DAIRY-FREE · GLUTEN-FREE · LOW FIBER · LOW FODMAP

Pho is a soothing, gluten-free Vietnamese rice noodle soup. This version is made with simple ingredients and comes together in no time.

1 teaspoon ground ginger

¼ teaspoon ground cinnamon

¼ teaspoon ground nutmeg

1 (32-ounce) container chicken, beef, or vegetable stock

4 cups water

1 tablespoon onion- or shallot-infused olive oil

1 tablespoon garlic-infused olive oil

½ pound protein of your choice (leftover chicken, raw beef, raw shrimp, or tofu), cut into bite-size pieces

8 ounces vermicelli rice noodles

Optional toppings

Chopped fresh cilantro

Fresh basil

Lime juice

Soy sauce

1. In a large stockpot over medium heat, toast the ginger, cinnamon, and nutmeg for 1 to 3 minutes, until the spices are fragrant.

2. Add the stock, water, and onion- and garlic-infused oils to the pot and bring the broth to a simmer.

3. Cover and allow the broth to simmer for 30 minutes.

4. Add your protein of choice to the broth and cook for 5 minutes (until the beef is cooked through or the shrimp are opaque and pink in color).

5. Add the rice noodles and cook for 2 minutes.

6. Serve each bowl of pho with your choice of toppings.

make it milder: This recipe uses flavor-infused olive oils, which add flavor to the broth without high-FODMAP onions or garlic. Infused olive oils are low FODMAP.

Per Serving: Calories: 640; Total Fat: 27g; Saturated Fat: 13g; Total Carbohydrates: 40g; Fiber: 1g; Sugars: 0g; Protein: 14g

Bone Broth

PREP TIME 15 MINUTES ✻ **COOK TIME** 13 TO 24 HOURS, PLUS 1 HOUR TO COOL
MAKES 16 CUPS

FLARE-UP · REMISSION · DAIRY-FREE · GLUTEN-FREE · LOW FAT · LOW FIBER · LOW FODMAP

Bone broth is a nourishing soup that contains no solids, making it both easy to digest and soothing to eat. The collagen and amino acids are healing to the gut, and the minerals will help restore nutrients that may have been lost during a flare-up.

2 tablespoons olive oil
2 pounds beef
  marrow bones

1 pound carrots, peeled and
  coarsely chopped
½ cup apple cider vinegar

1 tablespoon ground ginger
1 tablespoon ground
  turmeric

1. Preheat the oven to 400°F. Line a baking sheet with foil.
2. Rub the olive oil all over the marrow bones and place them on the prepared baking sheet.
3. Roast the bones in the oven for 1 hour.
4. Put the roasted bones, carrots, vinegar, ginger, and turmeric into a 6-quart slow cooker.
5. Add just enough water to cover the ingredients.
6. Cook on low for at least 12 hours, but ideally 24 hours, adding water as needed to keep the bones covered.
7. Using a slotted spoon, remove the bones from the broth and discard them.
8. Strain the broth and discard the solids.

9. Allow the broth to cool for up to 1 hour. Skim the fat off the top of the broth and discard it.

10. Portion the broth into mason jars or other storage containers; store it in the refrigerator for 3 to 4 days, or freeze it for up to 1 year.

substitution: If you do not benefit from this beef bone broth, you can make it with chicken bones, but the breakdown of the cartilage will result in a high-FODMAP broth. Your system may prefer one variation over the other.

ingredient tip: You can purchase marrow bones at the butcher counter of your local grocery store or butcher shop. If you are using chicken bones, you can simply use the leftover carcass of a whole chicken you have cooked and eaten at home.

Per Serving (1 cup): Calories: 38; Total Fat: 2g; Saturated Fat: 0g; Total Carbohydrates: 5g; Fiber: 1g; Sugars: 3g; Protein: 1g

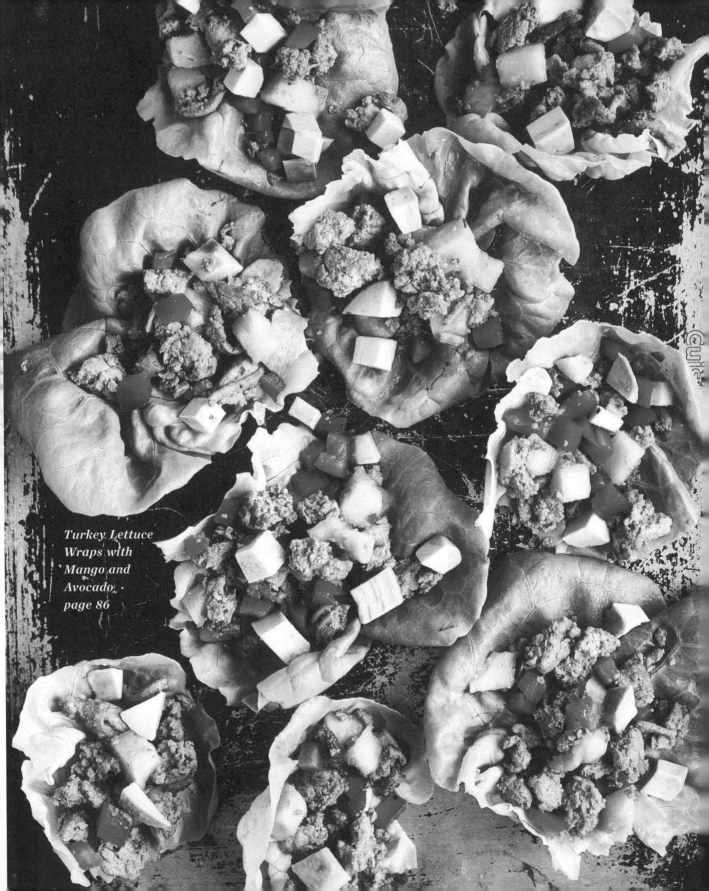

Turkey Lettuce Wraps with Mango and Avocado · page 86

CHAPTER 6

Salads

Raise your hand if you have been afraid to enjoy a salad while living with Crohn's disease. This may be because leafy green salads are full of fiber, which can cause a great deal of discomfort for someone with Crohn's, or it may be that the cheese- and dairy-based dressings do not agree with you. Shying away from salads is completely understandable; however, all of the salads in this chapter are Crohn's-friendly, in addition to providing a variety of textures, flavors, and nutrients.

Fruit Salad

PREP TIME 20 **MINUTES** ⨝ **SERVES** 4

FLARE-UP · REMISSION · DAIRY-FREE · GLUTEN-FREE · LOW FAT · LOW FIBER · PALEO

This fruit salad is full of Crohn's-friendly fruit, delivering vibrant flavor plus essential vitamins and minerals. It makes a great side dish with any meal or a refreshing dessert.

2 tablespoons lime juice

1 tablespoon honey

½ cantaloupe, cut into bite-size pieces

½ honeydew melon, cut into bite-size pieces

1 apple, peeled and cut into bite-size pieces

2 bananas, sliced

1 mango, peeled, pitted, and cut into bite-size pieces

1 tablespoon minced fresh mint, for garnish

1. In a small bowl, whisk together the lime juice and honey.
2. In a large bowl, combine all the fruit, then pour in the lime-honey dressing and gently toss.
3. Serve with the fresh mint as garnish.

make it milder: Knowing your unique system, feel free to vary the fruits in this recipe to make it work for your body.

make it easier: Use the leftovers from this recipe to make smoothies. Simply put the prepared salad in a blender and puree until smooth.

Per Serving: Calories: 227; Total Fat: 1g; Saturated Fat: 0g; Total Carbohydrates: 58g; Fiber: 6g; Sugars: 46g; Protein: 3g

Avocado-Cucumber Salad

PREP TIME 20 MINUTES ❊ **SERVES** 2 TO 4

FLARE-UP · REMISSION · DAIRY-FREE · GLUTEN-FREE · LOW FIBER · LOW FODMAP · PALEO

This lettuce-free salad can be served alone, in a wrap or sandwich, or over rice or pasta. This recipe makes enough for two main dishes or four side dishes.

2 cucumbers, peeled, seeded, and cut into ½-inch dice

1 large avocado, cut into ½-inch dice

¼ cup chopped scallions, green parts only, or minced fresh chives

2 tablespoons finely minced parsley or cilantro

1 tablespoon garlic-infused olive oil

1 tablespoon lime juice

1 tablespoon lemon juice

Salt

1. In a large bowl, combine all the ingredients.
2. Cover and refrigerate for 10 minutes to let the flavors combine.
3. Serve chilled.

ingredient tip: An avocado is ripe when the skin is purple to black, with little to no green, and it yields to gentle pressure. If it feels firm, it is not ripe yet, and if it feels mushy, it is overly ripe.

Per Serving: Calories: 75; Total Fat: 5g; Saturated Fat: 1g; Total Carbohydrates: 7g; Fiber: 3g; Sugars: 2g; Protein: 2g

Warm Potato Salad

PREP TIME 10 MINUTES ✖ COOK TIME 25 MINUTES, PLUS 5 MINUTES TO COOL
SERVES 4

FLARE-UP · REMISSION · DAIRY-FREE · GLUTEN-FREE · LOW FIBER · LOW FODMAP

Potato salad is a backyard barbeque favorite. This warm European-style potato salad is a healthier and easier-to-digest version, with an olive oil dressing instead of mayonnaise.

2 pounds potatoes, peeled and cut into bite-size pieces
1 hard-boiled egg, crumbled
½ cup diced scallions, green parts only, or minced fresh chives

1 tablespoon Dijon mustard
1 tablespoon olive oil
1 tablespoon white wine vinegar

1 tablespoon minced fresh dill
1 tablespoon minced fresh basil
Salt

1. Fill a medium stockpot or saucepan ¾ of the way with water and bring to a boil.

2. Add the potatoes and boil for 15 to 20 minutes, until the potatoes are tender when pierced with a fork.

3. Drain the water and set the potatoes aside to cool for 5 minutes.

4. In a large bowl, combine the cooked potatoes with the remaining ingredients, and toss until well combined.

5. Sprinkle with salt and serve.

substitution: If you're craving a creamy potato salad, substitute nondairy yogurt for the olive oil and vinegar.

ingredient tip: Red potatoes are traditional in potato salad, but they can be time consuming to peel. Yukon Gold, russet, or Idaho potatoes may be easier to work with.

Per Serving: Calories: 220; Total Fat: 5g; Saturated Fat: 1g; Total Carbohydrates: 39g; Fiber: 5g; Sugars: 2g; Protein: 6g

Veggie-Potato Salad

PREP TIME 15 MINUTES ✖ COOK TIME 30 MINUTES, PLUS 15 MINUTES TO CHILL
SERVES 4
FLARE-UP · REMISSION · DAIRY-FREE · GLUTEN-FREE · LOW FAT · LOW FIBER · LOW FODMAP · PALEO

This potato salad is full of easy-to-digest carbohydrates, as well as vitamin-rich squash. The flavors are crisp and bright without being weighed down by mayonnaise. This dish can be eaten as a vegetarian main dish or a side dish, warm or chilled.

1 Yukon Gold potato, peeled and cut into bite-size pieces

1 sweet potato or yam, peeled and cut into bite-size pieces

1 yellow squash, peeled, seeded, and chopped

1 zucchini, peeled, seeded, and chopped

¼ cup unsweetened plain nondairy yogurt

2 tablespoons Dijon mustard

1 tablespoon finely chopped fresh chives or scallions, for garnish

1. In a large stockpot over medium-high heat, combine the potato and sweet potato and cover with water. Bring to a boil.

2. Boil for 20 to 30 minutes, until the potatoes are tender when pierced with a fork.

3. Drain and transfer the potatoes to a large bowl.

4. Refrigerate the potatoes for 10 to 15 minutes.

5. Add the squash, zucchini, yogurt, and mustard. Mix the ingredients together until they are well combined.

6. Serve with a garnish of chives.

make ahead: You can make this potato salad in advance and leave it in the refrigerator overnight or for a couple of hours, which lets the flavors meld together.

Per Serving: Calories: 92; Total Fat: 1g; Saturated Fat: 1g; Total Carbohydrates: 19g; Fiber: 3g; Sugars: 5g; Protein: 3g

Vegetable-Quinoa Salad

PREP TIME 15 MINUTES ✳ **COOK TIME** 20 MINUTES, PLUS 10 MINUTES TO COOL
SERVES 4

REMISSION · DAIRY-FREE · GLUTEN-FREE · LOW FAT · LOW FODMAP

I have included butter lettuce in some of these recipes because it is easy to digest, it's a great source of vitamins and minerals, and it makes a fresh addition to the meal, but feel free to skip it if it doesn't agree with you.

1 cup water
½ cup quinoa, rinsed
1 carrot, peeled and
　shredded

½ yellow bell pepper, peeled
　and cut into ½-inch dice
½ mango, peeled, pitted,
　and cut into ½-inch dice
1 tablespoon olive oil

1 tablespoon white
　wine vinegar
½ head butter lettuce,
　shredded or torn

1. In a medium saucepan, bring the water to a boil.
2. Add the quinoa, reduce the heat to low, and cover the pot. Cook the quinoa for 15 minutes or until it can be fluffed with a fork.
3. Allow the quinoa to cool for 10 minutes.
4. In a large bowl, combine the quinoa, carrot, bell pepper, mango, oil, and vinegar, and stir until all ingredients are evenly distributed.
5. Serve over a bed of butter lettuce.

make it milder: This warm salad would also work well with white rice in place of quinoa, if quinoa does not sit well on your gut.

Per Serving: Calories: 147; Total Fat: 5g; Saturated Fat: 1g; Total Carbohydrates: 23g; Fiber: 3g; Sugars: 9g; Protein: 4g

Pasta Salad

PREP TIME 10 MINUTES ✻ **COOK TIME** 15 MINUTES, PLUS 20 MINUTES TO COOL
SERVES 4

FLARE-UP · REMISSION · DAIRY-FREE · LOW FIBER · LOW FODMAP · PALEO

A cold pasta salad is a great way to vary your diet with textures and flavors that are different from warm pasta dishes. This recipe uses nondairy yogurt in place of mayonnaise for a lower-fat, low-FODMAP variation that still tastes great.

4 quarts water

1 (16-ounce) box small pasta, like ditalini or small shells

1 (4.25-ounce) can sliced black olives, drained

1 zucchini or cucumber, peeled, seeded, and cut into ½-inch dice

2 hard-boiled eggs, crumbled

½ cup plain unsweetened nondairy yogurt

½ teaspoon ground thyme

1 teaspoon dried oregano

1. In a medium stockpot or saucepan, bring 4 quarts of water to a boil.

2. Add the pasta and boil for 8 to 12 minutes, until it is tender.

3. Drain the pasta and set it aside to cool for 5 minutes.

4. In a large bowl, toss the cooked pasta with the remaining ingredients until they are well combined.

5. Cover and place the pasta salad in the refrigerator for 15 minutes to cool.

6. Serve as an entrée or alongside your meal.

substitution: If gluten is a trigger for you, you can make this recipe with your favorite gluten-free pasta.

make ahead: This recipe stores easily in the refrigerator for up to 4 days, and the flavors get even better when it is served as leftovers.

Per Serving: Calories: 265; Total Fat: 9g; Saturated Fat: 1g; Total Carbohydrates: 37g; Fiber: 5g; Sugars: 2g; Protein: 12g

Chicken Salad Wraps

PREP TIME 10 MINUTES ❖ **SERVES** 2

FLARE-UP · REMISSION · DAIRY-FREE · LOW FIBER · PALEO

Chicken salad is often prepared as a mayonnaise-based comfort food. The fat content in mayonnaise can be triggering for people with Crohn's, but this Dijon mustard–based dressing is safe to eat—and more flavorful.

1 cup chopped or shredded cooked chicken or canned chicken

1 apple, peeled and cut into bite-size pieces

2 tablespoons Dijon mustard

1 tablespoon olive oil

1 tablespoon lemon juice

½ teaspoon ground cinnamon

2 white flour tortillas

1. In a medium bowl, combine the chicken, apple, mustard, olive oil, lemon juice, and cinnamon. Mix until the chicken and apples are coated with the dressing.
2. Serve each tortilla with half of the chicken salad mixture.

substitution: Half a diced avocado would work well in this recipe, providing additional healthy fat and creaminess. You can also use butter lettuce as wraps instead of tortillas if you prefer.

Per Serving: Calories: 440; Total Fat: 16g; Saturated Fat: 4g; Total Carbohydrates: 50g; Fiber: 6g; Sugars: 13g; Protein: 26g

Chicken Cobb Salad

PREP TIME 15 MINUTES ⋇ SERVES 2 TO 4

REMISSION · DAIRY-FREE · GLUTEN-FREE · LOW FIBER · LOW FODMAP · PALEO

A classic chicken Cobb salad includes blue cheese crumbles, bacon, and a cream-based dressing. This Crohn's-friendly variation does not skimp on flavor, but dismisses the digestive upset.

4 cups chopped butter lettuce
1 avocado, diced
2 hard-boiled eggs, crumbled
1 cup chopped or shredded cooked chicken
1 Roma tomato, peeled and seeded
1 tablespoon white wine vinegar
1 tablespoon olive oil
1 tablespoon Dijon mustard

1. In a large bowl, toss all the ingredients together until well combined.
2. Serve as an entrée or alongside a rice or pasta side dish.

make it milder: Omit the chicken from this recipe and add an extra egg if chicken is sitting heavily on your system.

make ahead: This recipe makes a great mason-jar salad, dressing and all, to build in advance and grab on the go.

Per Serving: Calories: 235; Total Fat: 14g; Saturated Fat: 3g; Total Carbohydrates: 5g; Fiber: 3g; Sugars: 1g; Protein: 23g

Sweet Potato–Quinoa Chicken Salad

PREP TIME 15 MINUTES ⁜ **COOK TIME** 1 HOUR ⁜ **SERVES** 4

REMISSION · DAIRY-FREE · GLUTEN-FREE · LOW FODMAP

Sweet potatoes are a good source of vitamins A, C, and B_6, as well as potassium. Even better, sweet potatoes are rich in antioxidants and reduce inflammation. Quinoa is a high-protein whole grain that adds a nutty flavor and chewy texture that is different from rice.

1 tablespoon canola oil

½ pound boneless, skinless chicken breast, cut into bite-size pieces

2 cups chicken stock

½ teaspoon ground cinnamon

½ cup quinoa, rinsed

1 sweet potato, peeled and cut into ½-inch dice

2 cups chopped butter lettuce (optional)

1. In a large stockpot over medium-high heat, heat the oil until shimmering.
2. Add the cubed chicken and cook for 5 to 7 minutes, until cooked through.
3. Add the chicken stock and cinnamon and bring to a boil.
4. Add the quinoa and sweet potato, then simmer for 20 to 30 minutes, until the sweet potato is tender and the quinoa can be fluffed with a fork.
5. Most of the liquid should have cooked off, but you can allow the mixture to steam for a few more minutes until most of the liquid has evaporated.
6. Allow the mixture to cool for 10 minutes.
7. Serve as it is or over butter lettuce, if desired.

make it milder: Quinoa is well tolerated by many people with Crohn's, but if it is hard on your system, feel free to omit it or use rice instead.

make it easier: This recipe can also be made in a slow cooker. Simply put all the ingredients into the slow cooker and cook on high for 3 to 4 hours. Serve over butter lettuce.

Per Serving: Calories: 210; Total Fat: 6g; Saturated Fat: 1g; Total Carbohydrates: 21g; Fiber: 3g; Sugars: 3g; Protein: 16g

Taco Salad

PREP TIME 15 MINUTES ※ **SERVES** 2 TO 4

REMISSION · DAIRY-FREE · GLUTEN-FREE · LOW FIBER · LOW FODMAP · PALEO

When you think of a taco salad, you might think of a deep-fried tortilla shell filled with a tiny bit of lettuce and a few veggies, then piled high with meat, cheese, and sour cream. This taco salad is just as delicious, but much healthier and gentler to eat.

1 tablespoon garlic-infused olive oil

1 tablespoon lime juice

¼ teaspoon ground cinnamon

1 teaspoon dried oregano

½ head butter lettuce, shredded

1 cup chopped or shredded cooked chicken

1 (4.25-ounce) can sliced black olives, drained

1 avocado, cut into ½-inch dice

½ bell pepper, peeled and cut into ½-inch dice

1 medium tomato, peeled and seeded

1 tablespoon unsweetened plain nondairy yogurt (optional)

1. In a small bowl, whisk together the oil, lime juice, cinnamon, and oregano.
2. In a large bowl, toss together the lettuce, chicken, olives, avocado, bell pepper, and tomato.
3. Serve with a drizzle of dressing and a dollop of nondairy yogurt, if desired.

substitution: If beans sit well with your system, ¼ cup to ½ cup black or pinto beans per serving would make a delicious addition to this taco salad.

ingredient tip: To peel a tomato, use a vegetable peeler or sharp paring knife and work back and forth in a sawing motion to get under the thin skin.

Per Serving: Calories: 247; Total Fat: 16g; Saturated Fat: 2g; Total Carbohydrates: 6g; Fiber: 3g; Sugars: 2g; Protein: 20g

Turkey Lettuce Wraps with Mango and Avocado

PREP TIME 15 MINUTES ✖ **COOK TIME** 15 MINUTES ✖ **SERVES** 4

REMISSION · DAIRY-FREE · LOW FIBER · PALEO

A 2017 study from Texas A&M University found that IBD patients showed positive digestive benefits from eating mango. Mangos are a particularly good source of polyphenols called gallotannins, which are highly anti-inflammatory.

½ pound 93% lean ground turkey

1 mango, peeled, pitted, and cut into ½-inch dice

½ avocado, cut into ½-inch dice

1 red bell pepper, peeled and cut into ½-inch dice

1 teaspoon soy sauce

1 tablespoon lime juice

1 teaspoon dried oregano

8 to 12 butter lettuce leaves

1. Line a plate with a paper towel.
2. In a medium skillet, brown the turkey over medium heat, which should take about 15 minutes.
3. Transfer the turkey to the paper-towel-lined plate to drain any excess fat.
4. Put the drained turkey in a large bowl.
5. Add the diced mango, avocado, and bell pepper and mix well.
6. Add the soy sauce, lime juice, and oregano and toss to coat.
7. Serve in butter lettuce leaf "wraps."

make it milder: To enjoy this recipe during a flare-up, try it without the butter lettuce, or try the wrap without the turkey. You know your body best!

Per Serving: Calories: 211; Total Fat: 10g; Saturated Fat: 2g; Total Carbohydrates: 17g; Fiber: 3g; Sugars: 13g; Protein: 17g

Tuna Salad

PREP TIME 10 MINUTES ✳ **SERVES** 2

REMISSION · DAIRY-FREE · GLUTEN-FREE · LOW FAT · LOW FIBER · LOW FODMAP · PALEO

Tuna salad is a staple in the American lunch box. The fatty fish is both anti-inflammatory and full of omega-3 fatty acids. Swapping out the mayonnaise for olive oil and some seasonings lightens this tuna salad, making it easier on the digestive system.

1 (5-ounce) can chunk light tuna, drained

½ carrot, peeled and shredded

1 celery stalk, finely minced

½ tablespoon olive oil

1 teaspoon lemon juice

1 teaspoon dried dill

⅛ teaspoon ground or dried thyme

1. In a medium bowl, mix all the ingredients until they are well combined.
2. Serve on crackers, soft bread, or butter lettuce.

make it milder: Replace the raw carrots and celery with leftover cooked carrots or celery, or try canned carrots, since the softer vegetables will be easier to digest.

substitution: You can use unsweetened plain nondairy yogurt in place of the olive oil and lemon juice for a mayonnaise-like dressing.

Per Serving: Calories: 104; Total Fat: 4g; Saturated Fat: 1g; Total Carbohydrates: 3g; Fiber: 1g; Sugars: 1g; Protein: 18g

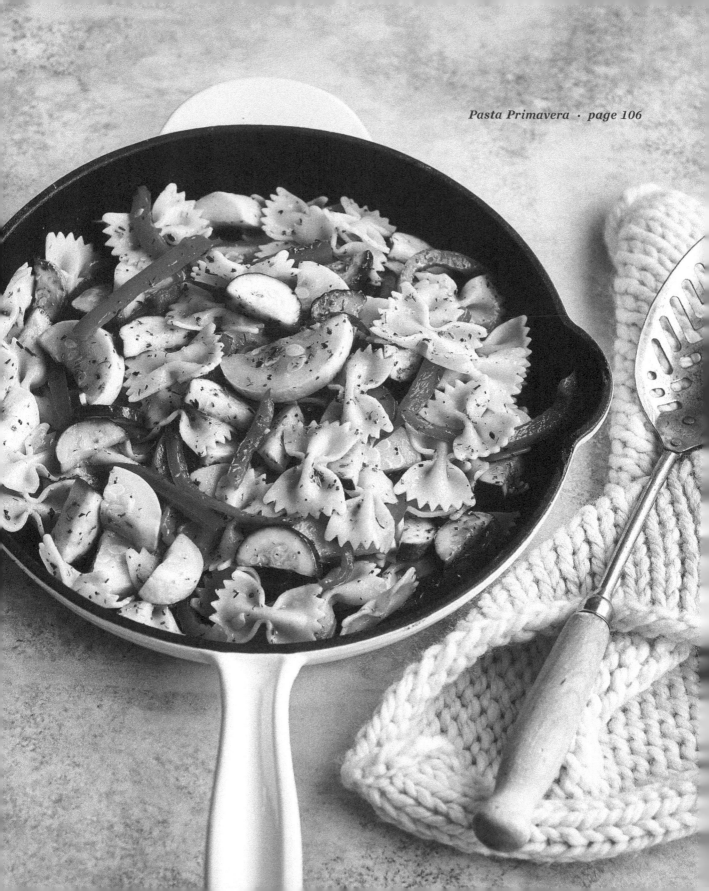

Pasta Primavera · *page 106*

CHAPTER 7

Vegetarian

Cooked vegetables are an excellent source of important vitamins and minerals that are also gentle on your gut. This chapter has a variety of recipes that prove vegetables still belong in a Crohn's diet.

Baked Potato Bar

PREP TIME 5 MINUTES ✳ COOK TIME 1 HOUR
1 POTATO PER PERSON

FLARE-UP · REMISSION · DAIRY-FREE · GLUTEN-FREE · LOW FAT ·
LOW FIBER (IF NO POTATO SKIN) · LOW FODMAP

Potatoes have nutrient-dense skin and tender, mildly sweet flesh. Although they are mainly made up of carbohydrates, potatoes also contain protein and are an excellent source of potassium, vitamins B_6 and C, and folate. Potatoes, especially red and purple varieties, also contain polyphenols, a type of antioxidant.

1 russet potato per person

Topping ideas:
Olive oil and salt
Plain unsweetened
  nondairy yogurt

Sliced avocado
Minced fresh herbs
  including parsley, cilantro,
  and dill
Finely chopped scallions or
  fresh chives

Marinara sauce with peeled,
  seeded, and chopped
  zucchini, heated together
Barbeque sauce

1. Preheat the oven to 425°F.

2. Scrub the potatoes under running water to remove any sediment.

3. Pat the potatoes dry. Do not rub the potatoes with any oil or wrap them in foil. This will allow you to easily remove the skin if needed.

4. Bake the potatoes for 45 to 60 minutes. A small potato will cook faster than a large potato. The potatoes are done when they can be easily pierced with a fork.

5. To serve, add toppings of your choosing and enjoy. If you find potato skins do not bother your system, feel free to eat them with your meal. If you find the skins harsh, simply cut the baked potato in half, use potholders or paper towels to protect your hands, and squeeze the flesh out of the skin.

make it easier: Did you know you can cook a potato in the microwave? Pierce the potato with a fork a few times so steam can escape, and microwave it on high for 5 minutes.

Per Serving: Calories: 168; Total Fat: 0g; Saturated Fat: 0g; Total Carbohydrates: 39g; Fiber: 3g; Sugars: 1g; Protein: 5g

Spaghetti Squash

PREP TIME 5 MINUTES ⚜ COOK TIME 40 MINUTES, PLUS 10 MINUTES TO COOL
SERVES 2 TO 4

FLARE-UP · REMISSION · DAIRY-FREE · GLUTEN-FREE · LOW FAT · LOW FIBER · LOW FODMAP · PALEO

Spaghetti squash is unique from its squash cousins in that it has a stringy texture and, when scraped with a fork, turns into "noodles" that can be used as a substitute for pasta. Use this as a base for any sauce or toppings that suit you, whenever you are craving pasta but want nutrient-rich vegetables in its place.

1 large spaghetti squash

2 tablespoons olive oil

Salt

1 tablespoon chopped fresh parsley

1. Preheat the oven to 400°F. Line a baking sheet with foil.
2. Cut the spaghetti squash in half lengthwise and scoop out the seeds.
3. Massage each half of the squash with 1 tablespoon of olive oil and a sprinkle of salt.
4. Place the squash cut-side down on the prepared baking sheet and pierce it several times with a fork.
5. Roast the squash in the preheated oven for 40 minutes.
6. Remove the squash from the oven and allow it to cool for 5 to 10 minutes, or until it can be handled safely.
7. Use a fork to shred the inside of the squash to create the noodles. You can shred all the way down to the skin, which you will discard.
8. Sprinkle each plate of spaghetti squash with fresh parsley and salt.
9. Serve as a main dish with olive oil or tomato sauce, or as a vegetable side dish.

ingredient tip: If it sits well with you, Parmesan cheese goes well with spaghetti squash. Because it is very low in lactose, many people with lactose intolerance do well eating it.

Per Serving: Calories: 201; Total Fat: 9g; Saturated Fat: 2g; Total Carbohydrates: 31g; Fiber: 5g; Sugars: 13g; Protein: 3g

Zucchini Boats

PREP TIME 10 MINUTES ⁂ **COOK TIME** 40 MINUTES ⁂ **SERVES** 2 TO 4

FLARE-UP · REMISSION · DAIRY-FREE · GLUTEN-FREE · LOW FAT · LOW FIBER · LOW FODMAP

Zucchini boats are a hearty, filling, refreshing meal that won't make you feel overly full or uncomfortable. This tasty version is stuffed with rice and mushroom sauce, which creates a delightful, meaty texture.

½ cup water

¼ cup rice

2 zucchini

½ cup finely chopped button mushrooms

1 (8-ounce) can tomato sauce

¼ teaspoon dried basil

¼ teaspoon dried oregano

¼ teaspoon salt

1. In a small saucepan over high heat, bring the water to a boil.
2. Add the rice, cover the pot, reduce the heat to low, and cook the rice for 15 to 20 minutes, until all the water has been absorbed.
3. Preheat the oven to 400°F. Line a baking sheet with foil.
4. While the rice is cooking, peel the zucchini, cut them in half lengthwise, and then scoop out and discard the seeds.
5. In a medium bowl, combine the cooked rice, mushrooms, tomato sauce, basil, oregano, and salt.
6. Fill each zucchini half with one-quarter of the mushroom-rice mixture.
7. Place the zucchini boats faceup on the prepared baking sheet.
8. Cover the baking sheet with foil, and bake the zucchini boats for 20 minutes.
9. Serve warm.

ingredient tip: You can also leave the zucchini peels on and scoop the flesh from the boats as you eat, leaving the skins to discard.

Per Serving: Calories: 54; Total Fat: 1g; Saturated Fat: 0g; Total Carbohydrates: 10g; Fiber: 3g; Sugars: 5g; Protein: 3g

Stuffed Pumpkins

PREP TIME 15 MINUTES ⁘ **COOK TIME** 1 HOUR ⁘ **SERVES** 2 TO 4

FLARE-UP · REMISSION · DAIRY-FREE · GLUTEN-FREE · LOW FAT · LOW FIBER

Pumpkins are not just for your Thanksgiving pie. They are vitamin-rich, flavorful squash that are easy to digest, so you can enjoy this soothing and savory recipe during either a flare-up or remission.

2 small pie or sugar
    pumpkins, rinsed
2 tablespoons olive oil
2 cups button
    mushrooms, washed

4 cups chopped
    fresh spinach
¼ cup brown sugar or honey
¼ teaspoon ground thyme

½ teaspoon ground
    cinnamon
½ teaspoon ground nutmeg

1. Preheat the oven to 350°F. Line a baking sheet with parchment paper.
2. Cut the top off each pumpkin and discard the tops.
3. Using a large spoon or melon baller, remove the seeds and strings from the inside of the pumpkins, just like if you were carving jack-o'-lanterns.
4. Place the pumpkins cut-side down on the prepared baking sheet, and bake for 45 minutes.
5. Meanwhile, in a large bowl, combine the oil, mushrooms, spinach, brown sugar, thyme, cinnamon, and nutmeg until the vegetables are evenly coated with the oil, sugar, and spices.
6. After the first bake, remove the pumpkins from the oven and carefully turn them cut-side up using tongs or hot pads.
7. Fill each pumpkin with half of the mushroom-spinach mixture.
8. Return the pumpkins to the oven and bake for 15 more minutes.
9. To enjoy the pumpkins, eat the flesh and vegetable stuffing from the inside, leaving the skin to be discarded.

substitution: This recipe would also work with acorn squash if pumpkins are not available.

Per Serving: Calories: 359; Total Fat: 8g; Saturated Fat: 1g; Total Carbohydrates: 72g; Fiber: 7g; Sugars: 39g; Protein: 12g

Ratatouille

PREP TIME 20 MINUTES ⁘ **COOK TIME** 1 HOUR ⁘ **SERVES** 4

FLARE-UP · REMISSION · DAIRY-FREE · GLUTEN-FREE · LOW FAT · LOW FIBER · LOW FODMAP · PALEO

Ratatouille is not just an animated film about a rat chef. It is also a stewed vegetable dish from the south of France featuring a wide variety of vegetables. Squash, peppers, eggplant, tomato, and onion are common ingredients.

Nonstick cooking spray, for greasing the pan

1 (15-ounce) can crushed tomatoes, drained

1 (15-ounce) can tomato sauce

1 teaspoon dried basil

½ teaspoon dried thyme

1 orange bell pepper, peeled and sliced into ⅛-inch-thick rings

1 eggplant, peeled and sliced into ⅛-inch-thick rounds

1 yellow squash, peeled, seeded, and sliced into ⅛-inch-thick rounds

2 tablespoons olive oil

1. Preheat the oven to 350°F. Lightly coat the inside of a 9-inch cake pan with nonstick cooking spray.
2. In a small bowl, mix the tomatoes, tomato sauce, basil, and thyme. Pour the mixture into the cake pan.
3. Working from the outside in, layer alternating slices of each vegetable in concentric circles, until you have filled the pan with spirals of vegetables. Brush the vegetables with the olive oil.
4. Cover the pan with foil and roast in the oven for 45 minutes.
5. Remove the foil and roast for 15 more minutes.
6. Serve with a spoonful of the pan sauce on top.

make it easier: Ratatouille does not have to be a pretty or fancy dish. You can also simply dice the vegetables and cook them in a pot like a stew.

Per Serving: Calories: 174; Total Fat: 8g; Saturated Fat: 1g; Total Carbohydrates: 26g; Fiber: 9g; Sugars: 16g; Protein: 5g

Veggie Pitas

PREP TIME 10 MINUTES, PLUS 10 MINUTES TO MARINATE ✕ **SERVES** 4

FLARE-UP · REMISSION · DAIRY-FREE · LOW FAT · LOW FIBER · LOW FODMAP

Pita is a Mediterranean flatbread often stuffed with delicious fillings or dipped into smooth sauces. This recipe is packed with flavor and can be made from pantry staples, making it a quick and inexpensive meal.

1 beefsteak tomato, peeled, seeded, and sliced

1 cucumber, peeled, seeded, and sliced

¼ cup black or kalamata olives, pitted

1 tablespoon olive oil

2 teaspoons red wine vinegar

1 teaspoon lemon juice

1 tablespoon dried or fresh chopped basil

¼ teaspoon ground thyme

4 pita pockets

1. In a large bowl, toss together the tomato, cucumber, olives, oil, vinegar, lemon juice, basil, and thyme. Allow the vegetables to marinate for 10 minutes.

2. Fill each pita with some of the veggies, drizzle with any dressing remaining in the bowl, and serve.

make it easier: You can use any vegetables you have on hand in these simple pitas.

Per Serving: Calories: 201; Total Fat: 7g; Saturated Fat: 1g; Total Carbohydrates: 30g; Fiber: 5g; Sugars: 4g; Protein: 8g

Vegetable Paninis

PREP TIME 1 HOUR ⁂ COOK TIME 30 MINUTES, PLUS 10 MINUTES TO STEAM ⁂ SERVES 4

FLARE-UP · REMISSION · DAIRY-FREE · LOW FAT · LOW FIBER · LOW FODMAP

A panini is a crunchy, comforting toasted sandwich. The tofu has a mozzarella-like feel. Complete with roasted red peppers and mild spices, this is sure to become a new favorite.

14 ounces extra-firm tofu

2 tablespoons tomato paste

1 tablespoon lemon juice

½ tablespoon dried oregano

1 teaspoon ground turmeric

¼ teaspoon salt

4 slices white bread

2 red bell peppers, cut in half and seeded

4 slices white bread

½ avocado, sliced

2 tablespoons olive oil

1. Line a plate with a thick stack of paper towels, and place the block of tofu on top.

2. Put additional paper towels on top of the tofu, then place a cutting board on top of the paper towels.

3. Weight the cutting board down with a heavy book, pot, or several cans.

4. Leave the tofu to be pressed for at least 30 minutes.

5. Cut the tofu into 4 slices.

6. In a large bowl, whisk together the tomato paste, lemon juice, oregano, turmeric, and salt.

7. Put the tofu in the tomato paste mixture and marinate it for 30 minutes.

8. Preheat the oven to 400°F. Line a baking sheet with foil.

9. Place the marinated tofu and bell peppers on the prepared baking sheet and roast them for 20 minutes, flipping after 10 minutes.

10. Remove the bell peppers from the oven and place them in a large sandwich bag. Allow the peppers to steam for 5 to 10 minutes to loosen their skins.

11. While the peppers steam, brush the bread with olive oil and broil it in the oven for 2 to 4 minutes, watching carefully to prevent burning.

12. Run the bell pepper under cold water and peel the skins off.

13. Build each panini with the white bread, a slice of tofu, half a roasted bell pepper, and half the avocado slices. Brush the bread with the olive oil and toast in the oven (still on broil) for 2 minutes per side. Serve warm.

substitution: Use your favorite gluten-free bread to make this recipe gluten-free.

make it easier: To save time, you can purchase canned fire-roasted peppers. Be sure to check the ingredients to make sure they are not too spicy or filled with garlic or onions.

Per Serving: Calories: 299; Total Fat: 18g; Saturated Fat: 3g; Total Carbohydrates: 23g; Fiber: 4g; Sugars: 6g; Protein: 17g

Veggie Burgers

PREP TIME 10 MINUTES ✻ **COOK TIME** 30 MINUTES ✻ **SERVES** 4

FLARE-UP · REMISSION · DAIRY-FREE · LOW FAT · LOW FIBER · LOW FODMAP

Many veggie burgers rely on beans or lentils as their base, but these foods can cause gas and discomfort, especially for someone with digestive sensitivity. These burgers are bean-free, making them completely Crohn's-friendly.

1 cup water

½ cup white rice

1 zucchini, peeled, seeded, and shredded

1 (15-ounce) can sweet potato puree or 1¾ cups mashed sweet potatoes or yams

1 cup bread crumbs or 4 pieces of toasted bread, crumbled

2 eggs, beaten

2 teaspoons dried oregano

1 teaspoon ground turmeric

½ teaspoon salt

Nonstick cooking spray, for greasing the skillet

4 white hamburger buns

2 leaves butter lettuce, for topping

1 avocado, sliced, for topping

1. In a medium saucepan over high heat, bring the water to a boil.

2. Add the rice, cover the pot, reduce the heat to low, and leave it to cook for 15 to 20 minutes, until all the water has been absorbed.

3. Place the shredded zucchini into a large square of paper towels and wring the excess moisture out.

4. In a large bowl, combine the cooked rice, zucchini, sweet potato puree, bread crumbs, eggs, oregano, turmeric, and salt.

5. Lightly coat the inside of a large skillet with nonstick cooking spray, and place the skillet over medium heat.

6. Form one-quarter of the rice-vegetable mixture into a patty. Repeat with the remaining mixture to make four patties.

7. Place the patties in the hot skillet and cook for 4 to 5 minutes per side, until browned.

8. Build each burger on a bun with butter lettuce, avocado, and the condiments of your choosing.

make it easier: You can save stale bread or leftover rice if you are planning on making these burgers as part of your weekly meal plan.

make ahead: You can make a larger batch of these burgers, stack them with a square of parchment paper between each one, and store them in a freezer-safe bag or container for up to 6 months.

Per Serving: Calories: 411; Total Fat: 5g; Saturated Fat: 1g; Total Carbohydrates: 78g; Fiber: 7g; Sugars: 11g; Protein: 14g

"Everything" Tofu

PREP TIME 1 HOUR ⋇ **COOK TIME 40 MINUTES** ⋇ **SERVES 2 TO 4**

FLARE-UP · REMISSION · DAIRY-FREE · LOW FAT · LOW FIBER · LOW FODMAP · PALEO

Tofu is an easy-to-digest protein that absorbs flavors beautifully. Make a batch of this marinated tofu and use it in dishes throughout the week. You can use it in just about anything.

14 ounces extra-firm tofu

1 tablespoon low-sodium soy sauce

1 tablespoon honey

1 tablespoon lemon juice

1 teaspoon ground ginger

1. Line a plate with a thick stack of paper towels, and place the block of tofu on top.
2. Put additional paper towels on top of the tofu, then place a cutting board on top of the paper towels.
3. Weight the cutting board down with a heavy book, pot, or several cans.
4. Leave the tofu to be pressed for at least 30 minutes.
5. Preheat the oven to 350°F. Line a baking sheet with parchment paper.
6. Cut the tofu into 1-inch cubes.
7. In a large bowl, whisk together the soy sauce, honey, lemon juice, and ginger.
8. Add the tofu and marinate for 30 minutes.
9. Place the tofu on the prepared baking sheet in a single layer.
10. Bake for 20 minutes, turn the cubes, and bake for 20 minutes more.
11. Serve with salad, pasta, or roasted vegetables, or eat the tofu as a snack.

substitution: Make this recipe gluten-free by substituting tamari for the soy sauce.

Per Serving: Calories: 130; Total Fat: 7g; Saturated Fat: 1g; Total Carbohydrates: 7g; Fiber: 1g; Sugars: 5g; Protein: 14g

Tofu Stir-Fry

PREP TIME 1 HOUR ✖ **COOK TIME** 15 MINUTES ✖ **SERVES** 4

REMISSION · DAIRY-FREE · LOW FAT · LOW FIBER · LOW FODMAP · PALEO

Making a stir-fry is a great opportunity to experiment with vegetables and proteins that work well for you. I have shared my favorite combination here, but feel free to experiment with flavors and foods that you like.

14 ounces extra-firm tofu

1 tablespoon soy sauce

1 tablespoon honey

1 tablespoon lemon juice

1 teaspoon ground ginger

2 tablespoons olive oil

1 red bell pepper, peeled and cut into ½-inch dice

1 cup peeled and shredded carrots

1 (8-ounce) can water chestnuts, drained

1. Line a plate with a thick stack of paper towels, and place the block of tofu on top.

2. Put additional paper towels on top of the tofu, then place a cutting board on top of the paper towels.

3. Weight the cutting board down with a heavy book, pot, or several cans. Leave the tofu to be pressed for at least 30 minutes.

4. Cut the tofu into 1-inch cubes.

5. In a large bowl, whisk together the soy sauce, honey, lemon juice, and ginger.

6. Add the tofu and marinate for 30 minutes.

7. In a large skillet or wok, heat the olive oil over medium heat.

8. Stir-fry the tofu, bell pepper, carrots, and water chestnuts for 5 to 10 minutes.

9. Serve over your favorite noodles or rice, or by itself if you follow a paleo diet.

substitution: Make this recipe gluten-free by substituting tamari for the soy sauce.

make it easier: You do not have to press the water out of the tofu. The texture of the tofu will be softer and the dish will have more liquid, but it's okay to skip if you're short on time.

Per Serving: Calories: 224; Total Fat: 12g; Saturated Fat: 2g; Total Carbohydrates: 20g; Fiber: 4g; Sugars: 7g; Protein: 12g

Burrito Bowls

PREP TIME 5 MINUTES ✄ **COOK TIME** 20 MINUTES ✄ **SERVES** 2 TO 4

FLARE-UP · REMISSION · DAIRY-FREE · GLUTEN-FREE · LOW FAT · LOW FIBER · LOW FODMAP · PALEO

Build-your-own burrito restaurants are a popular fast-casual option. Making burrito bowls at home gives you the freedom to customize them to your unique needs and avoid any trigger foods.

2 cups water

1 cup white rice

1 tablespoon canola oil, divided

¼ cup chopped fresh cilantro

2 tablespoons lime juice

½ teaspoon salt

1 (14.5-ounce) can diced tomatoes, drained

1 avocado, sliced

2 tablespoons plain unsweetened nondairy yogurt (optional)

White flour tortillas (optional)

1. In a medium saucepan over high heat, combine the water, rice, and ½ tablespoon of the oil.

2. Bring the rice to a boil, then reduce the heat to low, cover the pot, and cook for 15 to 20 minutes, until all the water has been absorbed.

3. Add the chopped cilantro, lime juice, salt, and remaining oil, and stir together until all the ingredients are well incorporated.

4. Build a burrito bowl with cilantro-lime rice on the bottom, and layer with diced tomatoes, avocado, and a dollop of nondairy yogurt as a substitute for sour cream, if desired.

5. Serve with tortillas (optional).

substitution: If dairy does not bother you, this is a great recipe to add cheese or sour cream to for some extra calcium. Also, if beans do not bother you, ¼ cup per serving would add protein to these bowls.

ingredient tip: The oil in this recipe prevents the rice from sticking together, so it stays fluffy in the refrigerator.

Per Serving: Calories: 282; Total Fat: 9g; Saturated Fat: 1g; Total Carbohydrates: 46g; Fiber: 5g; Sugars: 3g; Protein: 5g

Vegetable Enchiladas

PREP TIME 10 **MINUTES** ※ **COOK TIME** 30 **MINUTES** ※ **SERVES** 4

FLARE-UP · REMISSION · DAIRY-FREE · LOW FAT · LOW FIBER

Mexican food is often missed on a food plan for Crohn's, but no longer! With some simple swaps, you can enjoy traditional Mexican dishes like enchiladas without the tummy trouble.

- 1 avocado, cut into ½-inch dice
- ½ mango, peeled, pitted and cut into ½-inch dice
- 1 tablespoon lime juice
- 1 (15-ounce) can fire-roasted diced tomatoes, drained
- ½ tablespoon dried oregano
- 2 zucchini, peeled, seeded, and cut into ½-inch dice
- 1 cup finely chopped mushrooms
- 1 tablespoon garlic-infused olive oil
- 12 (6-inch) flour tortillas
- 1 (4.25-ounce) can sliced black olives, drained
- Plain unsweetened nondairy yogurt (optional)

1. Preheat the oven to 350°F. Set out an 8-by-8-inch baking dish.
2. In a small bowl, combine the avocado, mango, and lime juice. Mix well.
3. In a separate small bowl, combine the diced tomatoes and oregano; mix well.
4. In a large bowl, mix the zucchini, mushrooms, and olive oil.
5. Lay out the flour tortillas, and fill each one with about ½ cup of the zucchini-mushroom mixture.
6. Roll the tortillas up and nestle them closely together in the baking dish, seam-side down.
7. Cover the enchiladas with the diced tomato mixture.
8. Bake the enchiladas for 30 minutes.
9. Serve the enchiladas with the avocado-mango salsa, black olives, and a dollop of nondairy yogurt.

make ahead: Enchiladas make a great leftover meal, but they tend to fall apart a bit, so consider your leftovers to be more of a casserole.

Per Serving: Calories: 705; Total Fat: 26g; Saturated Fat: 5g; Total Carbohydrates: 101g; Fiber: 19g; Sugars: 14g; Protein: 19g

Pad Thai

Pad Thai is a noodle dish that is both savory and sweet. The creamy peanut butter in this recipe gives it a luscious texture and delicious peanut flavor without adding crunchy nuts on top. The eggs give the pasta a boost of easy-to-digest protein.

1 quart water

6 ounces pasta, like spaghetti or linguine

2 tablespoons natural creamy peanut butter

2 tablespoons white vinegar or rice vinegar

1 tablespoon soy sauce

2 tablespoons canola oil

2 large eggs, beaten

2 tablespoons chopped scallions, green parts only, or minced fresh chives

Lime juice (optional)

1. In a medium stockpot over high heat, bring the water to a boil.

2. Add the pasta and cook for 8 to 10 minutes, until tender.

3. Meanwhile, in a small bowl, whisk together the peanut butter, vinegar, and soy sauce.

4. Drain the pasta and return it to the pot.

5. Create a well in the middle of the pasta by pushing it to the edges of the pot.

6. Pour the oil into the well and heat it over medium heat until shimmering.

7. Pour the beaten eggs into the well and slowly stir them until small curds begin to form.

8. Stir the scrambled egg into the pasta.

9. Add the peanut butter sauce and stir well to combine all the ingredients.

10. Top with the scallions and lime juice, if desired, and serve.

substitution: You can substitute sunflower seed butter or tahini for the peanut butter, depending on which your system likes best. Also, to make this recipe gluten-free, you can use rice noodles and omit the soy sauce or substitute it for tamari.

make ahead: This recipe reheats well, so you can make a larger batch and save some for later in the week.

Per Serving: Calories: 267; Total Fat: 19g; Saturated Fat: 3g; Total Carbohydrates: 16g; Fiber: 3g; Sugars: 1g; Protein: 10g

Pasta Primavera

PREP TIME 10 MINUTES ⚒ **COOK TIME** 20 MINUTES ⚒ **SERVES** 4

FLARE-UP · REMISSION · DAIRY-FREE · LOW FAT · LOW FIBER · LOW FODMAP

Pasta primavera sounds very Italian, but it is an American dish inspired by Italian and American flavors. At its core, it is a pasta dish with fresh vegetables—a simple way to use up vegetables you have sitting in the fridge. It makes for a quick, easy, and tasty meal.

2 quarts water
8 ounces pasta, any shape
2 tablespoons olive oil

1 yellow squash, peeled, seeded, and sliced into half-moons
1 zucchini, peeled, seeded, and sliced into half-moons

1 red bell pepper, peeled and sliced into strips
1 tablespoon herbes de Provence
Lemon juice

1. In a large stockpot over high heat, bring the water to a boil.
2. Add the pasta and cook for 8 to 12 minutes, until tender.
3. Meanwhile, in a large, deep skillet, heat the olive oil over medium heat.
4. Cook the squash, zucchini, and bell pepper for 3 to 5 minutes, until they begin to soften.
5. Drain the pasta and add it to the vegetables.
6. Add the herbes de Provence and mix with tongs until all the ingredients are evenly coated in oil and herbs.
7. Serve with a squeeze of lemon juice.

make it milder: This recipe calls for fresh vegetables. To make the vegetables easier to digest, cook them for 5 more minutes to soften them further.

ingredient tip: You can make your own Herbs de Provence spice blend at home by mixing equal proportions of dried thyme, marjoram, rosemary, sage, and fennel seed.

Per Serving: Calories: 169; Total Fat: 9g; Saturated Fat: 1g; Total Carbohydrates: 21g; Fiber: 4g; Sugars: 3g; Protein: 5g

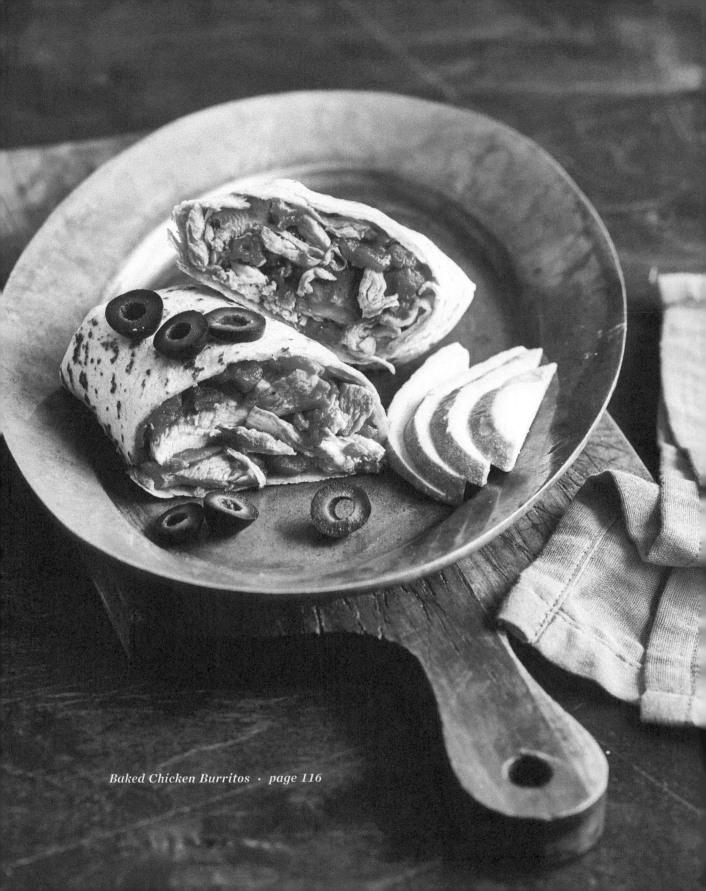

Baked Chicken Burritos · page 116

CHAPTER 8

Meat & Poultry

Meat is an efficient source of important nutrients like protein and vitamin B_{12}. However, large quantities of meat, especially red meat, take more work to digest, which can place an extra burden on the digestive system. Fear no more. This collection of meat and poultry recipes is full of dishes that aren't just delicious, but are also tender and easy to digest.

Lemon Chicken

PREP TIME 10 MINUTES ⁑ **COOK TIME** 7 TO 8 HOURS ON LOW, 3 TO 4 HOURS ON HIGH
SERVES 4 WITH LEFTOVERS

FLARE-UP · REMISSION · DAIRY-FREE · GLUTEN-FREE · LOW FAT · LOW FIBER · LOW FODMAP · PALEO

This slow-cooker recipe is about to become one of your busy day go-tos. The slow-cooking process allows the lemon and herbs to fully penetrate the chicken and potatoes, leaving them tender and bursting with flavor when served.

1 pound boneless, skinless chicken breast

4 Yukon Gold or yellow potatoes, peeled and halved

1 (32-ounce) container chicken stock

1 tablespoon dried oregano

1 tablespoon dried basil

1 teaspoon ground turmeric

4 lemons, halved and seeded

1. Put the chicken, potatoes, stock, oregano, basil, and turmeric in a slow cooker.
2. Squeeze in the lemon juice and drop in the squeezed lemon halves.
3. Cook on low for 7 to 8 hours or on high for 3 to 4 hours.
4. Remove the lemon halves and discard.
5. Serve the chicken and potatoes with a generous spoonful of the cooking liquid.

make it milder: To enjoy some protein without aggravating your system, serve yourself a plate with more of the flavorful potatoes and less chicken.

make ahead: This recipe makes a good amount of leftovers, which can be stored in the refrigerator for 3 to 4 days and easily reheated in the microwave.

Per Serving: Calories: 278; Total Fat: 4g; Saturated Fat: 1g; Total Carbohydrates: 34g; Fiber: 4g; Sugars: 3g; Protein: 29g

Chicken and Eggs

PREP TIME 10 MINUTES ※ COOK TIME 10 MINUTES ※ SERVES 2 TO 4

REMISSION · DAIRY-FREE · GLUTEN-FREE · LOW FIBER · LOW FODMAP · PALEO

A play on both steak and eggs and chicken-fried steak, this dish features just three main ingredients and can be eaten any time of day. My personal thought? Breakfast for dinner is always a winner!

1 tablespoon olive oil
6 ounces boneless, skinless chicken breast, cut into bite-size pieces
2 eggs, beaten
1 small apple, peeled and cut into bite-size pieces
½ teaspoon ground turmeric
1 tablespoon minced fresh parsley

1. In a medium pan or skillet over medium heat, heat the oil until shimmering.
2. Add the chicken and cook for 3 to 5 minutes, until it is cooked through.
3. Add the eggs, apple, and turmeric to the chicken breast and mix continuously for 3 to 5 minutes, until the eggs are cooked through.
4. Serve with fresh parsley.

make it easier: Save time by using leftover cooked chicken. Simply reheat it before moving to step 3.

Per Serving: Calories: 136; Total Fat: 7g; Saturated Fat: 1g; Total Carbohydrates: 6g; Fiber: 1g; Sugars: 4g; Protein: 13g

Chicken and Green Beans

PREP TIME 10 MINUTES ✖ **COOK TIME** 15 MINUTES ✖ **SERVES** 4

FLARE-UP · REMISSION · DAIRY-FREE · LOW FIBER · LOW FODMAP · PALEO

Sometimes the most delicious meals are the simplest. With just chicken, a can of green beans, and a few flavorful pantry staples, this meal is ready in under 30 minutes.

2 tablespoons garlic-infused olive oil, divided

8 ounces boneless, skinless chicken breast, cut into bite-size pieces

1 (15-ounce) can cut green beans, drained

1 cup beef stock

1 tablespoon soy sauce

½ teaspoon ground ginger

1. In a skillet over medium heat, heat 1 tablespoon of olive oil until shimmering.

2. Add the chicken and cook for 3 to 5 minutes, until it is opaque.

3. Add the green beans, beef stock, soy sauce, and ginger to the chicken and mix.

4. Cook for 10 minutes or until the chicken is cooked through and most of the liquid has evaporated.

5. Serve on its own or with your favorite rice, pasta, or bread.

ingredient tip: This recipe uses canned green beans for their soft texture and convenience. You can use fresh green beans; just be sure they are well cooked and soft to make them easier to digest. Also, this recipe uses beef stock, which adds a more robust flavor, but chicken stock or vegetable stock works as well.

Per Serving: Calories: 168; Total Fat: 9g; Saturated Fat: 1g; Total Carbohydrates: 8g; Fiber: 3g; Sugars: 4g; Protein: 16g

Soy-Ginger Chicken

PREP TIME 15 MINUTES ⚹ **COOK TIME** 20 MINUTES ⚹ **SERVES** 4

FLARE-UP · REMISSION · DAIRY-FREE · LOW FIBER · LOW FODMAP

From egg rolls to sesame chicken to sweet-and-sour pork, Chinese takeout is an American favorite. This recipe is a home-cooked, Crohn's-friendly version of one of these favorites.

2½ cups water, divided
1 cup white rice
2 tablespoons olive oil

8 ounces boneless, skinless chicken breast, cut into bite-size pieces
1 red bell pepper, peeled and sliced into strips

2 tablespoons soy sauce
1 tablespoon honey
1 teaspoon ground ginger

1. In a medium saucepan over high heat, bring 2 cups of water to a boil.
2. Add the rice, reduce the heat to low, cover the pot, and cook for 15 to 20 minutes, until all the water has been absorbed.
3. Meanwhile, in a medium skillet over medium heat, heat the olive oil until shimmering.
4. Add the chicken and bell pepper and cook for 5 to 7 minutes.
5. Meanwhile, in a small bowl, whisk together the soy sauce, remaining ½ cup water, honey, and ginger.
6. Pour the sauce into the pan with the chicken and bell pepper. Cook together for 3 to 5 minutes.
7. Serve on a bed of rice with a spoonful of pan sauce.

substitution: Make this recipe gluten-free by substituting tamari for the soy sauce.

Per Serving: Calories: 324; Total Fat: 9g; Saturated Fat: 1g; Total Carbohydrates: 44g; Fiber: 1g; Sugars: 6g; Protein: 17g

Turmeric Chicken and Potatoes

PREP TIME 10 MINUTES ✳ **COOK TIME 5 TO 6 HOURS ON LOW, 2 TO 3 HOURS ON HIGH**
SERVES 4 WITH LEFTOVERS

FLARE-UP · REMISSION · DAIRY-FREE · GLUTEN-FREE · LOW FAT · LOW FIBER · LOW FODMAP · PALEO

The chicken and potatoes in this simple but flavorful slow-cooker dish simmer in a robust yellow sauce. Turmeric, which is a gorgeous yellow color, is an anti-inflammatory powerhouse that lends itself well to savory preparations.

1 pound boneless, skinless chicken breast, cut into bite-size pieces

4 Yukon Gold or yellow potatoes, peeled and quartered

1 (32-ounce) container chicken stock

2 tablespoons garlic-infused olive oil

2 teaspoons ground turmeric

1 teaspoon dried basil

1. Put the chicken, potatoes, stock, oil, turmeric, and basil in a slow cooker.

2. Cook on low for 5 to 6 hours or on high for 2 to 3 hours.

3. Serve the chicken and potatoes with a generous spoonful of the cooking liquid.

make it milder: To enjoy some protein without aggravating your system, serve yourself more of the flavorful potatoes topped with a smaller amount of chicken.

make ahead: This recipe makes a good amount of leftovers, which will keep in the refrigerator for 3 to 4 days and can be reheated in the microwave.

Per Serving: Calories: 390; Total Fat: 13g; Saturated Fat: 2g; Total Carbohydrates: 35g; Fiber: 2g; Sugars: 5g; Protein: 34g

Root Vegetable–Chicken Bake

PREP TIME 10 MINUTES ❋ **COOK TIME** 25 MINUTES ❋ **SERVES** 4

FLARE-UP · REMISSION · DAIRY-FREE · GLUTEN-FREE · LOW FIBER · LOW FODMAP

Sheet-pan meals are some of the simplest to make and most comforting to eat. This recipe requires just six ingredients, some quick prep, and a short time in the oven. You'll be ready to eat in about 30 minutes.

8 ounces boneless, skinless chicken breast

1 sweet potato or yam, peeled and coarsely chopped

1 Idaho or russet potato, peeled and coarsely chopped

2 carrots, peeled and coarsely chopped

2 tablespoons garlic-infused olive oil

1 teaspoon ground ginger

1. Preheat the oven to 400°F. Line a baking sheet with foil.
2. Place the chicken breasts in the center of the baking sheet and surround them with the root vegetables.
3. In a small bowl, whisk together the oil and ginger.
4. Brush the olive oil mixture onto the chicken and root vegetables.
5. Bake for 15 minutes, turn the root vegetables, and bake for 10 more minutes or until the chicken has reached an internal temperature of 165°F.
6. Serve warm.

make it milder: Serve yourself less chicken and more root vegetables to make this dish milder on the digestive system.

make ahead: This recipe makes great leftovers, which will keep for 3 to 4 days in the refrigerator. Or, double the recipe and freeze for up to 4 months.

Per Serving: Calories: 211; Total Fat: 9g; Saturated Fat: 1g; Total Carbohydrates: 19g; Fiber: 3g; Sugars: 3g; Protein: 15g

Baked Chicken Burritos

PREP TIME 5 MINUTES ※ **COOK TIME** 30 MINUTES ※ **SERVES** 2 TO 4

REMISSION · DAIRY-FREE · LOW FIBER · LOW FODMAP

In my family, we call these "burradas"—no relation to burrata, the soft Italian cheese! This cross between a burrito and an enchilada is simple but flavorful.

2 tablespoons garlic-infused olive oil, divided

6 ounces boneless, skinless chicken breast, cut into bite-size pieces

1 (15-ounce) can diced tomatoes, drained

1 tablespoon dried oregano

2 large flour tortillas

2 tablespoons sliced black olives, for serving

½ avocado, sliced, for serving

1. Preheat the oven to 400°F. Line a 9-by-5-inch loaf pan with parchment paper.
2. In a medium skillet over medium heat, heat 1 tablespoon of the oil.
3. Add the chicken and cook for 3 to 5 minutes, until it is opaque.
4. Add the diced tomatoes and the oregano and stir.
5. Use the tortillas to build 2 burritos, using half of the mixture in each. Fold the left and right sides of the tortilla toward the center, then, starting with the side closest to you, tightly roll up the tortilla.
6. Place the burritos in the loaf pan, side by side, and brush with the remaining olive oil.
7. Bake the burritos for 15 to 20 minutes, until the tops are golden brown.
8. Serve warm with black olives and sliced avocado.

make ahead: You can easily freeze a pan of these burritos for up to 6 months. To reheat, put them in the microwave on high for 1 minute, flip, and microwave for 1 minute more, or heat them in a 225°F oven for 30 minutes.

Per Serving: Calories: 237; Total Fat: 13g; Saturated Fat: 2g; Total Carbohydrates: 19g; Fiber: 4g; Sugars: 3g; Protein: 13g

Chicken Enchilada Casserole

PREP TIME 10 MINUTES ⋇ **COOK TIME** 30 MINUTES ⋇ **SERVES** 2 TO 4 WITH LEFTOVERS

REMISSION · DAIRY-FREE · GLUTEN-FREE · LOW FIBER · LOW FODMAP

This casserole-style dish is a fun mash-up between enchiladas and lasagna, layering tortillas, chicken, and veggies. The precooked rotisserie chicken from the grocery store is a huge time-saver.

2 cups shredded cooked rotisserie chicken

1 yellow squash, peeled, seeded, and cut into ½-inch dice

1 (15-ounce) can fire-roasted tomatoes, drained

½ teaspoon ground cinnamon

¼ teaspoon salt

12 corn tortillas

1 tablespoon garlic-infused olive oil

1. Preheat the oven to 350°F.
2. In a large bowl, combine the chicken, squash, tomatoes, cinnamon, and salt; mix well.
3. In a 9-by-9-inch baking dish, layer 4 corn tortillas so they cover the bottom of the dish.
4. Add half of the chicken-and-vegetable filling, spreading it in an even layer.
5. Cover the filling with 4 more corn tortillas.
6. Add the remaining filling, again spreading it in an even layer.
7. Cover the filling with the last 4 corn tortillas.
8. Brush the top layer with the oil and cover with foil.
9. Bake for 30 minutes. Remove and serve by the spoonful.

make it milder: Swap the corn tortillas for flour tortillas to make this recipe lower in fiber and even milder.

make ahead: This recipe makes plenty of leftovers that can be reheated later in the week. After a quick 3 to 5 minutes in the microwave, leftovers are served.

Per Serving: Calories: 478; Total Fat: 29g; Saturated Fat: 7g; Total Carbohydrates: 40g; Fiber: 7g; Sugars: 4g; Protein: 17g

Chicken-Vegetable Lasagna

PREP TIME 20 MINUTES ❋ COOK TIME 45 MINUTES
SERVES 2 TO 4 WITH LEFTOVERS

REMISSION · DAIRY-FREE · LOW FIBER · LOW FODMAP

Not to be confused with the Chicken Enchilada Casserole (page 117), this is a traditional lasagna—but without the lactose-filled cheese. Savor the Italian-inspired flavors here, without the stomach upset.

1 tablespoon olive oil

8 ounces boneless, skinless chicken breast, cut into bite-size pieces

1 (28-ounce) can tomato sauce

2 tablespoons garlic-infused olive oil

1 tablespoon dried oregano

1 tablespoon minced fresh basil

1 zucchini, peeled, seeded, and cut into ½-inch dice

1 cup sliced button mushrooms

12 ounces oven-ready lasagna noodles (about 15 noodles)

1. Preheat the oven to 350°F.
2. In a medium skillet over medium heat, heat the oil until shimmering.
3. Add the chicken and cook for 3 to 5 minutes, until it is opaque.
4. In a large bowl, combine the chicken, tomato sauce, garlic-infused olive oil, oregano, basil, zucchini, and mushrooms. Mix well.
5. In a 9-by-12-inch baking dish, layer 5 noodles so they cover the bottom of the dish.
6. Add half of the chicken-and-vegetable filling, spreading it in an even layer.
7. Repeat steps 5 and 6 for the middle layer.

8. Cover the filling with the last 5 noodles.

9. Cover with aluminum foil and bake for 45 minutes.

10. Serve by the spoonful.

ingredient tip: Although lasagna noodles are traditional, you can use any shape of noodles in this recipe and call it a pasta bake. Or use your favorite gluten-free noodles for a gluten-free version.

make ahead: This recipe makes plenty of leftovers that can be reheated later in the week. After a quick 3 to 5 minutes in the microwave, leftovers are served.

Per Serving: Calories: 357; Total Fat: 14g; Saturated Fat: 2g; Total Carbohydrates: 40g; Fiber: 8g; Sugars: 10g; Protein: 22g

Turkey Meat Loaf Sliders

PREP TIME 15 MINUTES ✻ **COOK TIME** 1 HOUR ✻ **SERVES** 4

FLARE-UP · REMISSION · DAIRY-FREE · LOW FIBER · LOW FODMAP

This recipe is a fresh take on your mother's meat loaf. Using turkey instead of beef and mushrooms instead of onions, these meat loaf sliders are gentle on the system but still satisfying when you're craving comfort food.

1 pound 93% lean
   ground turkey
8 ounces button
   mushrooms,
   finely chopped

1 bunch fresh
   parsley, minced
1 tablespoon garlic-infused
   olive oil
1 tablespoon
   Worcestershire sauce

2 tablespoons ketchup
1 cup bread crumbs
⅓ cup chicken stock
2 eggs, beaten
8 sweet Hawaiian rolls

1. Preheat the oven to 350°F. Line a 9-by-5-inch loaf pan with parchment paper.

2. In a large bowl, combine the turkey, mushrooms, parsley, olive oil, Worcestershire sauce, ketchup, bread crumbs, chicken stock, and eggs. Using clean or gloved hands, mash the mixture together until all the ingredients are evenly distributed.

3. Pack the mixture into the loaf pan.

4. Bake the meat loaf for 1 hour.

5. Slice the meat loaf into 2-by-2-inch slices and serve on sweet Hawaiian rolls.

substitution: Ground chicken will work well in place of the ground turkey in this recipe, if you prefer.

Per Serving: Calories: 625; Total Fat: 25g; Saturated Fat: 7g; Total Carbohydrates: 60g; Fiber: 3g; Sugars: 13g; Protein: 44g

Shepherd's Pie

PREP TIME 10 MINUTES ✳ **COOK TIME** 40 MINUTES ✳ **SERVES 4 WITH LEFTOVERS**

FLARE-UP · REMISSION · DAIRY-FREE · GLUTEN-FREE · LOW FAT · LOW FIBER · LOW FODMAP · PALEO

What we commonly refer to as shepherd's pie—the version of this dish made with beef—is actually an English dish called cottage pie. True shepherd's pie is an Irish classic made with lamb. This recipe deviates from both by using ground turkey and sweet potatoes, but it is equally delectable.

2 quarts water

2 large sweet potatoes or yams, peeled and cut into ½-inch dice

1 tablespoon olive oil

1 pound 93% lean ground turkey

2 tablespoons butter substitute

4 tablespoons unsweetened plain nondairy milk

15 ounces green peas, fresh, frozen, or canned (drained)

1 (8-ounce) can tomato sauce

1 teaspoon Worcestershire sauce

½ teaspoon dried rosemary

1. Preheat the oven to 400°F.
2. In a large stockpot over high heat, bring the water to a boil.
3. Add the sweet potatoes and cook for 15 minutes or until they are tender when pierced with a fork.
4. Meanwhile, in a medium skillet over medium heat, heat the olive oil until shimmering.
5. Add the ground turkey and cook for 15 minutes.
6. Drain the sweet potatoes, leaving a few tablespoons of the starchy liquid for mashing.
7. Add the butter substitute and nondairy milk and mash the sweet potatoes until there are no lumps.

continued...

8. In a 9-by-9-inch baking dish, combine the turkey, peas, tomato sauce, Worcestershire sauce, and rosemary, stirring together until all ingredients are well incorporated.

9. Spread the mashed sweet potatoes over the turkey mixture.

10. Bake uncovered for 20 minutes.

11. Serve by the spoonful.

make ahead: This is a great recipe to prep ahead of time and freeze for whenever you need a quick meal. Freeze in freezer-safe containers for up to 6 months. To reheat, bake in an oven-safe dish for 1 hour at 400°F.

Per Serving: Calories: 508; Total Fat: 23g; Saturated Fat: 5g; Total Carbohydrates: 39g; Fiber: 9g; Sugars: 11g; Protein: 39g

Pork Tenderloin with Sweet Potatoes

PREP TIME 10 **MINUTES** ⁜ **COOK TIME** 40 **MINUTES, PLUS** 5 **MINUTES TO REST** ⁜ **SERVES** 4

REMISSION · DAIRY-FREE · LOW FIBER · LOW FODMAP

Pork is often a trigger for people with Crohn's disease, but this recipe has been included for anyone that pork works well for. You can easily substitute chicken for the pork if it works better for you.

2 large sweet potatoes or yams, peeled and cubed
2 tablespoons olive oil
½ teaspoon ground cinnamon, divided
8 ounces pork tenderloin
1 tablespoon soy sauce

1. Preheat the oven to 400°F. Line a baking sheet with foil.
2. In a large bowl or zip-top plastic bag, toss together the potatoes, oil, and ¼ teaspoon of the cinnamon.
3. Place the sweet potatoes on the prepared baking sheet in a single layer. Leave about a quarter of the pan empty—that's where you'll cook the pork.
4. Using a separate sheet of foil, create a boat by folding up the sides and edges for the pork to rest in. Place the pork in the foil boat, and place the boat in the reserved space on the baking sheet.
5. Cover the pork with the soy sauce and sprinkle with the remaining cinnamon.
6. Bake for 20 minutes, turn the sweet potatoes and pork, and bake for 15 to 20 minutes more, watching for burning. The pork will be done when it reaches an internal temperature of 145°F.
7. Remove the pan from the oven and allow the pork to rest for at least 5 minutes.
8. Slice the pork into medallions and serve with the sweet potatoes.

Per Serving: Calories: 247; Total Fat: 10g; Saturated Fat: 2g; Total Carbohydrates: 21g; Fiber: 3g; Sugars: 4g; Protein: 18g

Sticky Ginger Pork
with Broccoli

PREP TIME 10 MINUTES ※ **COOK TIME** 30 MINUTES ※ **SERVES** 4

REMISSION · DAIRY-FREE · LOW FIBER · LOW FODMAP

Ginger is a nourishing, fragrant spice to enjoy in abundance. Here, it is combined with pork and broccoli for a tasty take on takeout. The vitamins and minerals in the broccoli can be protective to the gut, and in small amounts, well-cooked broccoli is a nutrient-dense addition to your diet.

1 cup white rice

2 cups plus
   1 tablespoon water

2 tablespoons soy sauce

1 tablespoon white
   wine vinegar

2 tablespoons honey

1 teaspoon ground ginger

2 tablespoons canola oil

8 ounces pork tenderloin,
   cut into 1-inch medallions

1 cup chopped broccoli,
   fresh or frozen

1. In a colander or strainer, rinse the rice several times.

2. In a medium saucepan over high heat, combine the water and rice.

3. Cover the pot and bring the water to a boil, then reduce the heat to low and simmer for 15 minutes.

4. Remove the pot from the stove and let the rice sit, covered, for 15 more minutes.

5. Meanwhile, in a small bowl, whisk together the soy sauce, vinegar, honey, and ginger.

6. In a medium skillet over medium heat, heat the oil until shimmering.

7. Add the pork medallions to the pan, and sear each side for 1 minute.

8. Add the sauce to the pan, cover, and cook for 10 minutes, stirring occasionally to prevent the sauce from burning.

9. Add the chopped broccoli to the pan and stir it into the sauce.

10. Cover and cook for 10 to 15 minutes, stirring occasionally to prevent the sauce from burning, until the broccoli is tender. The pork will be done when it reaches an internal temperature of 145°F.

11. Serve the pork and broccoli on a bed of sticky rice with a spoonful of pan sauce.

substitution: This recipe would also be delicious with cubed tofu or chicken in place of the pork. You can make it gluten-free by substituting tamari for the soy sauce.

make it easier: This recipe includes instructions for making sticky rice. To save time, you can cook the rice normally or use boil-in-bag rice.

Per Serving: Calories: 338; Total Fat: 9g; Saturated Fat: 1g; Total Carbohydrates: 48g; Fiber: 1g; Sugars: 9g; Protein: 17g

Roast Beef

PREP TIME 10 MINUTES ✳ **COOK TIME** 7 TO 8 HOURS ON LOW, 3 TO 4 HOURS ON HIGH
SERVES 4

REMISSION · DAIRY-FREE · GLUTEN-FREE · LOW FIBER · LOW FODMAP

Beef is often a trigger for people with Crohn's disease, but this recipe has been included for anyone that beef works well for. The beef can easily be replaced with chicken if that is what works best for your body.

8 ounces beef roast, such as pot roast or chuck roast

2 Idaho or russet potatoes, peeled and quartered

2 carrots, peeled and coarsely chopped

2 celery stalks, coarsely chopped

1 tablespoon Dijon mustard

1 teaspoon ground thyme

1. Put the beef, potatoes, carrots, celery, mustard, and thyme in a slow cooker.

2. Add enough water to just cover the beef and vegetables.

3. Cook on low for 7 to 8 hours or on high for 3 to 4 hours.

4. Serve the beef and vegetables with a generous spoonful of the cooking liquid.

substitution: Boneless, skinless chicken breast is leaner than beef, and the cooking process is the same. However, to prevent foodborne illness, be sure the internal temperature of the chicken reaches 165°F.

Per Serving: Calories: 142; Total Fat: 1g; Saturated Fat: 1g; Total Carbohydrates: 29g; Fiber: 4g; Sugars: 5g; Protein: 6g

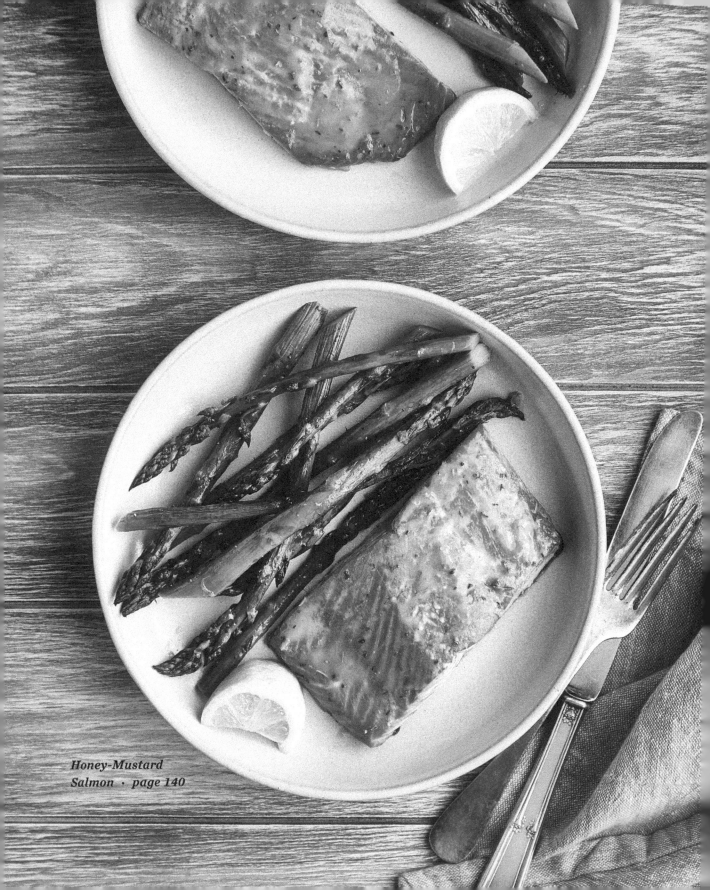

Honey-Mustard
Salmon · page 140

CHAPTER 9

Fish & Seafood

Fish and seafood are important in a food plan for Crohn's, since they are rich in anti-inflammatory omega-3 fatty acids, healthy unsaturated fats, B vitamins, and protein—and all easily digested. The variety of recipes in this chapter will have you craving seafood.

Shrimp Stir-Fry

PREP TIME 10 **MINUTES** ※ **COOK TIME** 10 **MINUTES** ※ **SERVES** 4

FLARE-UP · REMISSION · DAIRY-FREE · GLUTEN-FREE · LOW FAT · LOW FIBER · LOW FODMAP · PALEO

Bok choy is high in antioxidants and anti-inflammatory nutrients in the forms of selenium, vitamins C and E, and beta-carotene. It is also a low-FODMAP vegetable that is easier than most to digest, especially when cooked thoroughly.

2 tablespoons garlic-infused olive oil
1 carrot, peeled and grated
1 small head bok choy, coarsely chopped
8 ounces shrimp, peeled and deveined
1 zucchini, peeled, seeded, and chopped
½ tablespoon honey
1 tablespoon white wine vinegar
¼ teaspoon ground ginger

1. In a large skillet or wok over medium heat, heat the oil until shimmering.
2. Add the carrot and bok choy and cook for 5 minutes, until they start to soften.
3. Add the shrimp and zucchini and cook for 3 to 5 minutes, until the shrimp have turned pink.
4. Meanwhile, in a small bowl, whisk together the honey, vinegar, and ginger.
5. Add the sauce to the pan and stir-fry for 2 to 3 minutes.
6. Serve over your favorite rice or noodles, or on its own.

ingredient tip: If you are not comfortable cooking raw shrimp, you can purchase precooked shrimp at the grocery store seafood counter. Follow the same instructions to make sure the cooked shrimp are heated through.

Per Serving: Calories: 148; Total Fat: 8g; Saturated Fat: 1g; Total Carbohydrates: 10g; Fiber: 3g; Sugars: 7g; Protein: 11g

Ginger Shrimp with Sticky Rice

PREP TIME 10 MINUTES ✖ **COOK TIME** 30 MINUTES ✖ **SERVES** 4

FLARE-UP · REMISSION · DAIRY-FREE · GLUTEN-FREE · LOW FAT · LOW FIBER · LOW FODMAP

Shrimp can be cooked quite quickly (and flavorfully!) on the stove, due to their small size. Pairing them with a sweet ginger sauce and cooking them using this method will yield the flavor and texture that makes shrimp such a treat to eat.

1 cup white rice

2 cups water

2 tablespoons honey

1 teaspoon white wine vinegar

½ teaspoon ground ginger

8 ounces shrimp, peeled and deveined

1 tablespoon canola oil

1. In a colander or strainer, rinse the rice several times.
2. In a small pot over high heat, combine the water and rice.
3. Cover the pot and bring the rice to a boil, then reduce the heat to low and simmer for 15 minutes.
4. Remove the pot from the stove and let the rice sit, covered, for 15 more minutes.
5. Meanwhile, in a medium bowl, whisk together the honey, vinegar, and ginger.
6. Add the shrimp to the ginger sauce and coat them evenly.
7. In a medium skillet over medium heat, heat the oil until shimmering.
8. Cook the shrimp for 2 to 3 minutes per side, until they are pink in color.
9. Serve the shrimp on a bed of sticky rice.

make it easier: This recipe includes instructions for making sticky rice. To save time, you can cook the rice normally or use boil-in-bag rice. If you are not comfortable cooking raw shrimp, you can purchase precooked shrimp at the grocery store seafood counter. In step 8, simply cook them until they are heated through.

Per Serving: Calories: 288; Total Fat: 4g; Saturated Fat: 0g; Total Carbohydrates: 46g; Fiber: 1g; Sugars: 9g; Protein: 17g

Simple "Sushi" Bowls

PREP TIME 10 MINUTES ✳ SERVES 4

FLARE-UP · REMISSION · DAIRY-FREE · LOW FAT · LOW FIBER · LOW FODMAP

Sushi is something you might miss while living with Crohn's disease, because eating raw or undercooked proteins can be dangerous. Sushi is also difficult to make at home. This recipe solves both problems, using fully cooked fish and simple methods.

1 cup white rice

1½ cups water

¼ cup rice vinegar

½ tablespoon canola oil

2 tablespoons sugar

¼ teaspoon salt

1 cucumber, peeled, seeded, and diced

½ avocado, diced

4 ounces imitation crab or precooked shrimp

0.5 ounce seaweed crisps, crumbled

Soy sauce

1. In a colander or strainer, rinse the rice several times.

2. In a medium saucepan over high heat, combine the water and rice.

3. Bring the rice to a boil, then reduce the heat to low, cover, and simmer for 20 minutes.

4. Meanwhile, in a small saucepan, combine the vinegar, oil, sugar, and salt.

5. Cook the mixture over medium heat for 3 to 5 minutes, until the sugar and salt have fully dissolved.

6. Pour the mixture over the cooked rice, and stir until the rice has absorbed the liquid.

7. Build four "sushi" bowls by topping servings of rice with cucumber, avocado, imitation crab, crumbled seaweed crisps, and soy sauce to taste.

ingredient tip: You can find seaweed crisps at any grocer, usually in the international aisle near the Japanese products or in the snack aisle near the dried fruits and nuts.

make it easier: This recipe includes instructions for making sushi rice. To save time, you can cook the rice normally or use boil-in-bag rice.

Per Serving: Calories: 290; Total Fat: 5g; Saturated Fat: 1g; Total Carbohydrates: 54g; Fiber: 3g; Sugars: 9g; Protein: 6g

To Anchovy
(or Not to Anchovy) Pizza

PREP TIME 15 MINUTES ✻ **COOK TIME** 10 MINUTES ✻ **SERVES** 4

FLARE-UP · REMISSION · LOW FAT · LOW FIBER · LOW FODMAP

Anchovies are an oily saltwater fish rich in omega-3 fatty acids. They are also full of numerous vitamins and minerals, including the mineral selenium, a component of several antioxidants. These tiny fish fillets are packed with flavor, but this recipe includes a variation to omit them, since they are not everyone's favorite.

1 demi loaf soft French or
   Italian bread
2 tablespoons olive oil
1 (2-ounce) can flat anchovy
   fillets, drained (optional)

1 (8-ounce) can
   tomato sauce
½ tablespoon Italian
   seasoning

½ cup shredded
   mozzarella cheese
1 green bell pepper, peeled
   and sliced

1. Preheat the oven to broil or to 500°F. Line a baking sheet with foil.
2. Slice the bread in half lengthwise, then halve each half, making 4 pizza breads.
3. Brush the bread with the olive oil.
4. Finely mince the anchovies.
5. In a small bowl, combine the tomato sauce, Italian seasoning, and anchovies.
6. On the prepared baking sheet, toast the bread in the oven for 2 to 3 minutes, watching carefully to prevent burning.
7. Take the pan out of the oven and layer the pizza breads with the anchovy-tomato sauce, mozzarella cheese, and bell pepper.

continued...

8. Bake the pizza breads for 5 to 7 minutes, until the cheese has melted.
9. Serve warm.

substitution: It may seem odd to have pizza without cheese, but this dish is just as delicious without it. Feel free to omit the cheese or use a vegan cheese alternative.

Per Serving: Calories: 153; Total Fat: 11g; Saturated Fat: 3g; Total Carbohydrates: 11g; Fiber: 2g; Sugars: 3g; Protein: 6g

Sardine Patties

PREP TIME 10 MINUTES ✳ **COOK TIME** 10 MINUTES ✳ **SERVES** 4 WITH LEFTOVERS

REMISSION · DAIRY-FREE · LOW FIBER · LOW FODMAP

Sardines are an oily fish high in omega-3 fatty acids, calcium, iron, and B vitamins. You can buy sardines skinless and boneless, but both the skin and bones are edible, so it is completely up to your preference.

2 (4.4-ounce) cans sardines in water, drained
⅓ cup bread crumbs or crushed unsalted saltine crackers

1 egg
1 teaspoon lemon juice

1 teaspoon dried oregano
Nonstick cooking spray, for greasing the skillet

1. In a medium bowl, mash the sardines with a fork to achieve a flaked texture.
2. Add the bread crumbs, egg, lemon juice, and oregano.
3. With gloved or clean hands, blend the mixture thoroughly.
4. Form 4 patties.
5. Warm a large skillet over medium heat. Lightly coat the inside of the skillet with cooking spray.
6. Place the patties in the pan. Sear the patties for 3 to 5 minutes per side, until they reach your preferred level of crispiness.
7. Serve as a burger substitute on a bun, or as a protein entrée, with the condiments of your choice.

substitution: If you are not a sardine fan, you can substitute canned tuna or canned salmon for the sardines.

Per Serving: Calories: 176; Total Fat:8 g; Saturated Fat: 2g; Total Carbohydrates: 8g; Fiber: 1g; Sugars: 0g; Protein: 18g

Oven-Roasted Mackerel

PREP TIME 5 MINUTES ✳ **COOK TIME** 10 MINUTES ✳ **SERVES** 2

FLARE-UP · REMISSION · DAIRY-FREE · GLUTEN-FREE · LOW FIBER · LOW FODMAP · PALEO

Mackerel is an oily saltwater fish with a milder flavor than salmon. It's also less well known because it is harder to find in inland regions. Because mackerel is high in omega-3 fatty acids, it's perfect for eating with Crohn's—but if you cannot find it, salmon is a suitable substitute.

6 ounces boneless, skinless mackerel fillet

½ tablespoon lemon juice

2 tablespoons olive oil, divided

6 kalamata olives, pitted

6 pitted green olives, with or without pimentos

1 teaspoon dried or chopped fresh dill

1. Preheat the oven to broil or to 500°F.
2. Rub the mackerel with the lemon juice and 1 tablespoon of olive oil. Place it in a small baking dish.
3. Broil for 5 to 7 minutes, until the fillets begin to flake and they have reached an internal temperature of 145°F.
4. While the mackerel is cooking, finely chop the olives and mix them in a small bowl with the dill and remaining 1 tablespoon of olive oil.
5. Serve the mackerel with a generous spoonful of the olive tapenade.

ingredient tip: You can also cook mackerel in a skillet or on the grill over medium heat for 4 minutes per side.

Per Serving: Calories: 315; Total Fat: 26g; Saturated Fat: 4g; Total Carbohydrates: 3g; Fiber: 0g; Sugars: 0g; Protein: 22g

Fish Tacos

Tilapia is a mild, easily digested freshwater whitefish with a delicate flavor and texture. These tilapia tacos are gentle on your body and bright on the palate.

1 tablespoon garlic-infused olive oil
2 (6-ounce) tilapia fillets
1 teaspoon dried oregano

1 (15-ounce) can diced tomatoes, drained
½ avocado, cut into ½-inch dice

1 tablespoon lime juice
8 (6-inch) flour tortillas
2 leaves butter lettuce, shredded

1. In a medium skillet over medium heat, heat the oil until shimmering.
2. Sprinkle the tilapia fillets with the oregano and cook for 4 to 5 minutes per side, until the fish is opaque all the way through and flakes with a fork.
3. Meanwhile, in a medium bowl, mix the tomatoes, avocado, and lime juice.
4. Remove the tilapia from the pan and rest it on a paper-towel-lined plate while you warm the tortillas.
5. Wipe the pan with a paper towel and heat it over high heat.
6. Warm each tortilla for 1 minute per side.
7. Top the warm tortillas with tilapia, shredded lettuce, and the tomato-avocado salsa.

substitution: You can also use corn tortillas, which provide a sweetness and slight nuttiness.

Per Serving: Calories: 338; Total Fat: 16g; Saturated Fat: 2g; Total Carbohydrates: 39g; Fiber: 12g; Sugars: 3g; Protein: 20g

Lemony Trout

PREP TIME 15 MINUTES ✳ **COOK TIME** 10 MINUTES ✳ **SERVES** 4

FLARE-UP · REMISSION · DAIRY-FREE · GLUTEN-FREE · LOW FAT · LOW FIBER · LOW FODMAP · PALEO

Trout are freshwater fish high in omega-3 fatty acids, B vitamins, potassium, and phosphorus. They have a light pink flesh with a flavor similar to salmon, and they require only a simple preparation for full flavor. Fish skin, which is left on here, is a crispy treat that's full of omega-3s.

1 lemon, halved

2 brook trout, butterflied

¼ teaspoon salt

2 tablespoons olive oil

1. Thinly slice one half of the lemon. Juice the other half, and set the juice aside. Discard the rind.
2. Scale the trout by scraping the skin with a sharp knife against the grain of the scales. You can tell the scales are coming off when the skin has a "fishnet" look to it.
3. Thoroughly rinse the trout and pat them dry.
4. Place 2 lemon slices inside each trout, sprinkle with the salt, and fold the fish closed.
5. In a large sauté pan or skillet over medium heat, heat the oil until shimmering.
6. Panfry the trout on one side for 5 minutes, then flip and fry the other side for 5 minutes more. The fish is done cooking when it is opaque and easily flakes with a fork.
7. Serve with the fresh-squeezed lemon juice on top. You can leave the lemon slices inside the fish or remove them before eating.

ingredient tip: When you buy the trout at the fish counter, ask them to butterfly the fish for you. Even better, ask if they can scale them for you.

Per Serving: Calories: 123; Total Fat: 9g; Saturated Fat: 1g; Total Carbohydrates: 1g; Fiber: 0g; Sugars: 0g; Protein: 8g

Salmon-Avocado Wrap

PREP TIME 5 MINUTES ✴ **COOK TIME** 10 MINUTES ✴ **SERVES** 2 TO 4

FLARE-UP. REMISSION · DAIRY-FREE · LOW FIBER · LOW FODMAP

———————————

Some flavor pairings are classic, like peanut butter and jelly and butter and popcorn. Creamy dill sauce pairs perfectly here with salmon in the same harmonious way. As a bonus, the creamy dill sauce in this wrap is dairy-free.

1 tablespoon canola oil

6 ounces boneless, skinless salmon

1 tablespoon unsweetened plain nondairy yogurt

1 teaspoon lemon juice

1 teaspoon dried or chopped fresh dill

2 (10-inch or wrap-size) flour tortillas

2 leaves butter lettuce

½ avocado, sliced

1. In a medium skillet over medium heat, heat the oil until shimmering.

2. Sear the salmon for 3 to 4 minutes per side, until it flakes easily and the internal temperature has reached 145°F.

3. Meanwhile, in a small bowl, whisk together the yogurt, lemon juice, and dill.

4. On a microwave-safe plate, microwave the tortillas for 30 seconds to make them pliable.

5. Spread half of the dill sauce on each tortilla, then add the lettuce, avocado, and salmon.

6. Wrap tightly and serve.

substitution: Dijon mustard would work well in place of the creamy dill sauce.

———————————

Per Serving: Calories: 205; Total Fat: 11g; Saturated Fat: 2g; Total Carbohydrates: 16g; Fiber: 3g; Sugars: 1g; Protein: 12g

Honey-Mustard Salmon

PREP TIME 5 MINUTES ⌗ **COOK TIME** 15 MINUTES ⌗ **SERVES** 2

FLARE-UP · REMISSION · DAIRY-FREE · GLUTEN-FREE · LOW FIBER · LOW FODMAP · PALEO

Salmon is a fatty fish, rich in anti-inflammatory omega-3s, that works beautifully with both sweet and savory preparations. This recipe is both sweet and savory, featuring a honey-mustard glaze that caramelizes into a delicious coating while it bakes.

1 tablespoon Dijon mustard

1 tablespoon honey

1 teaspoon lemon juice

¼ teaspoon ground thyme

2 (3-ounce) boneless, skinless salmon fillets

1. Preheat the oven to 450°F. Line a small baking dish with foil.
2. In a small bowl, whisk together the mustard, honey, lemon juice, and thyme.
3. Pat the salmon dry and place it on the prepared baking dish.
4. Spread the honey-mustard mixture on the salmon.
5. Bake, uncovered, for 12 to 15 minutes, until the salmon reaches an internal temperature of 145°F.
6. Serve with rice, pasta, or vegetables.

ingredient tip: You can also panfry the salmon. Lightly coat the pan with cooking spray and cook for 4 minutes per side.

Per Serving: Calories: 218; Total Fat: 11g; Saturated Fat: 1g; Total Carbohydrates: 9g; Fiber: 0g; Sugars: 9g; Protein: 22g

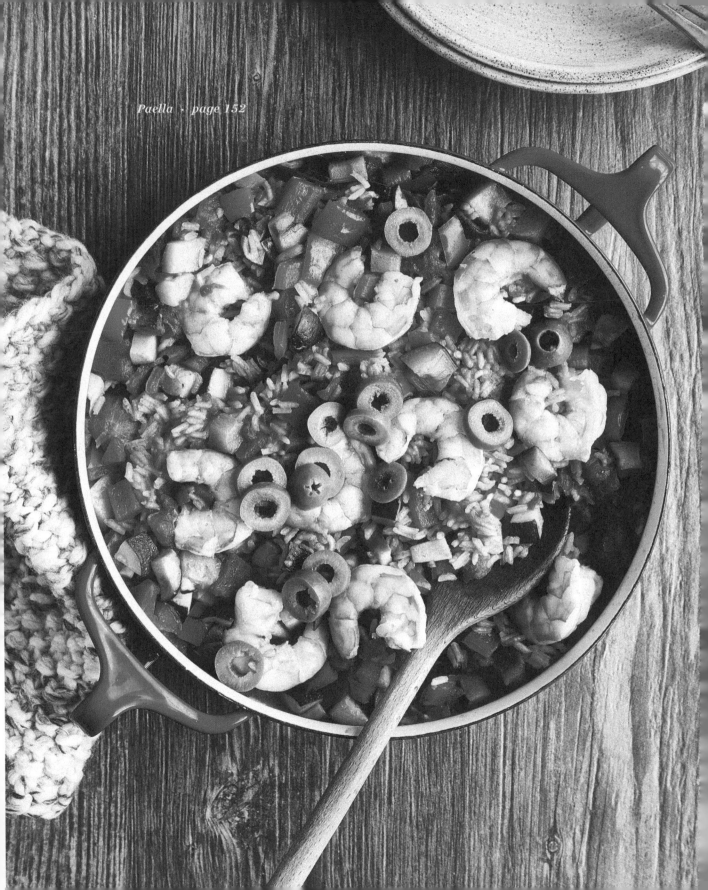

Paella · page 152

CHAPTER 10

Pasta & Rice

Pasta and rice are Crohn's staples that are easy to digest and quick to prepare. Grains make up a large part of our diets, providing valuable vitamins and minerals. Most importantly, they give us the calories our bodies and brains use as fuel.

Fried Rice

PREP TIME 5 MINUTES ✳ COOK TIME 20 MINUTES ✳ SERVES 2 TO 4

FLARE-UP · REMISSION · DAIRY-FREE · LOW FIBER · LOW FODMAP

Fried rice is a takeout favorite, but making it at home is almost as quick and easy as placing a to-go order. In under 30 minutes, you can have delicious fried rice anytime you want, for a fraction of the cost.

2 cups water

1 cup white rice

1½ tablespoons canola oil, divided

1 cup frozen or canned mixed vegetables (drain if canned)

2 large eggs, beaten

1 tablespoon soy sauce

1. In a medium saucepan over high heat, combine the water, rice, and ½ tablespoon of the oil.

2. Bring the rice to a boil, then reduce the heat to low, cover the pot, and cook for 15 to 20 minutes, until all the water has been absorbed.

3. In a skillet over medium heat, heat ½ tablespoon of the oil until shimmering; stir-fry the cooked rice with the mixed vegetables for 5 minutes.

4. Push the rice and vegetables to the edges of the pan to create a well in the middle.

5. Pour the remaining ½ tablespoon of oil into the well and heat until shimmering.

6. Pour the beaten eggs into the well, and stir the eggs until small curds begin to form.

7. Stir the scrambled eggs into the rice and vegetables.

8. Add the soy sauce and stir well to combine all the ingredients.

9. Serve warm.

ingredient tip: Short- and long-grain rice both work well in this recipe, as does jasmine rice. Whatever you have on hand is perfectly fine.

Per Serving: Calories: 255; Total Fat: 6g; Saturated Fat: 1g; Total Carbohydrates: 42g; Fiber: 2g; Sugars: 2g; Protein: 8g

Cranberry-Orange Rice

PREP TIME 10 MINUTES ✳ **COOK TIME** 20 MINUTES ✳ **SERVES** 2 TO 4

FLARE-UP · REMISSION · DAIRY-FREE · GLUTEN-FREE · LOW FAT · LOW FIBER · LOW FODMAP

Rice is a wonderful blank canvas to absorb flavor, and this bright, flavorful Thanksgiving-inspired rice is sure to become a year-round favorite. It makes for a wonderful side dish or base for the toppings of your choice.

1 cup plus
 1 tablespoon water
1 cup white rice

1 tablespoon orange zest
1 tablespoon cranberry jelly

1 teaspoon white
 wine vinegar
¼ teaspoon ground thyme

1. In a medium pot over high heat, bring the water and rice to a boil. Reduce the heat to low, cover the pot, and cook for 15 to 20 minutes, until all the water has been absorbed.

2. Meanwhile, in a small microwave-safe bowl, whisk together the orange zest, cranberry jelly, vinegar, and thyme.

3. Microwave the sauce for 30 seconds, stir, and set aside.

4. Pour the sauce over the cooked rice, stir well, and serve.

substitution: You can use orange juice in place of the orange zest if you prefer—or even lemon zest or lemon juice.

Per Serving: Calories: 178; Total Fat: 0g; Saturated Fat: 0g; Total Carbohydrates: 39g; Fiber: 1g; Sugars: 2g; Protein: 3g

Spinach Jasmine Rice

PREP TIME 5 MINUTES ✳ **COOK TIME** 25 MINUTES ✳ **SERVES** 2 TO 4

FLARE-UP · REMISSION · DAIRY-FREE · GLUTEN-FREE · LOW FAT · LOW FIBER · LOW FODMAP

Jasmine rice is a sticky type of rice with a sweet, floral aroma, but the type of rice you use is less important here. This recipe shows how you can get creative even with a pantry staple like rice.

1½ cups vegetable stock

1 cup jasmine rice

2 tablespoons water

1 tablespoon olive oil

2 cups fresh baby spinach, chopped

¼ teaspoon salt

Lemon juice

1. In a medium saucepan over high heat, bring the stock, rice, and water to a boil.
2. Reduce the heat to low, cover, and cook for 15 to 20 minutes, until all the water has been absorbed.
3. Remove the pot from the heat and leave covered for 5 minutes.
4. While the rice is cooling, heat the olive oil in a large skillet over medium heat until shimmering.
5. Add the spinach to the pan and cook for 5 minutes or until wilted.
6. Add the cooked rice and the salt to the spinach and mix until all ingredients are evenly distributed.
7. Serve with a squeeze of lemon juice.

ingredient tip: You can use short- or long-grain white rice in place of jasmine rice—the dish will just be slightly less aromatic. Also, you can use either fresh or frozen spinach in this preparation with minimal difference.

Per Serving: Calories: 79; Total Fat: 3g; Saturated Fat: 1g; Total Carbohydrates: 11g; Fiber: 0g; Sugars: 1g; Protein: 1g

Rice-Stuffed Squash

PREP TIME 10 MINUTES ✳ **COOK TIME** 45 MINUTES ✳ **SERVES** 4

FLARE-UP · REMISSION · DAIRY-FREE · GLUTEN-FREE · LOW FAT · LOW FIBER · LOW FODMAP

Unlike the other recipes in this chapter, this recipe is not rice- or pasta-centric. The flesh of the acorn squash gets so creamy and smooth that it acts as more of a sauce than a vegetable.

2 acorn squash, halved
  and seeded
4 tablespoons olive
  oil, divided

¼ teaspoon salt
2 cups plus 1 tablespoon
  chicken stock
1 cup rice

8 ounces mushrooms, sliced
2 tablespoons white
  wine vinegar

1. Preheat the oven to 400°F. Line a baking sheet with foil.

2. Rub the inside of the squash halves with 2 tablespoons of olive oil, and sprinkle with the salt.

3. Place the squash on the prepared baking sheet, cut-side down, and roast for 30 minutes.

4. Flip the squash over and roast for 15 more minutes.

5. Meanwhile, in a medium saucepan over high heat, bring the chicken stock and rice to a boil.

6. Reduce the heat to low, cover, and simmer for 15 to 20 minutes, until all the liquid has been absorbed.

7. While the rice cooks, in a large pan or skillet over medium heat, heat the remaining 2 tablespoons of oil until shimmering.

8. Add the mushrooms and cook for 3 minutes without stirring. Once the mushrooms start to brown, continue to cook for 3 to 5 more minutes, stirring periodically.

9. Add the cooked rice and vinegar to the mushrooms and stir.

continued...

10. When the squash halves have finished roasting, remove them from the oven and set 3 of them aside.

11. Scoop the flesh from the fourth squash half and mash it with a fork or potato masher until no lumps remain.

12. Stir the mashed squash into the rice and mushroom mixture until it is evenly distributed.

13. Fill each of the 3 remaining squash halves with a scoop of the rice and mushroom mixture.

14. To enjoy, scoop each bite from the center, until just the skin remains. The skin can be discarded.

ingredient tip: When grocery shopping, look for a good acorn squash; it will feel heavy and smooth with few blemishes.

make it easier: You can also roast or boil cubed acorn squash while the rice is cooking, and simply serve the rice and squash tossed together or alongside each other.

Per Serving: Calories: 396; Total Fat: 14g; Saturated Fat: 2g; Total Carbohydrates: 62g; Fiber: 8g; Sugars: 3g; Protein: 8g

Spanish Rice

PREP TIME 5 MINUTES ✕ **COOK TIME** 30 MINUTES ✕ **SERVES** 2 TO 4

FLARE-UP · REMISSION · DAIRY-FREE · GLUTEN-FREE · LOW FAT · LOW FIBER · LOW FODMAP

Living with Crohn's disease does not mean you have to give up your favorites. This Spanish rice is mild on the system but full of flavor.

1 tablespoon garlic-infused olive oil

1 cup rice

2 cups chicken stock

1 cup canned diced tomatoes, drained

1 tablespoon tomato paste

¼ teaspoon cumin

¼ teaspoon salt

1. In a large, deep skillet over medium heat, heat the olive oil until shimmering.

2. Add the rice and toast it in the oil for 3 to 5 minutes, stirring frequently to prevent burning.

3. Add the stock, tomatoes, tomato paste, cumin, and salt and stir.

4. Increase the heat to medium-high and bring the rice to a boil.

5. Reduce the heat to low, cover, and simmer for 15 to 20 minutes, until the rice is cooked through and can be fluffed with a fork.

6. Remove the lid and cook until all remaining liquid has evaporated, 5 to 10 minutes more.

7. Serve as a main dish or as a side.

make it easier: You do not have to toast the rice. To save time, you can skip steps 1 and 2.

Per Serving: Calories: 262; Total Fat: 5g; Saturated Fat: 1g; Total Carbohydrates: 45g; Fiber: 2g; Sugars: 4g; Protein: 7g

Étouffée

PREP TIME 15 MINUTES ※ COOK TIME 30 MINUTES ※ SERVES 2 TO 4

FLARE-UP · REMISSION · DAIRY-FREE · GLUTEN-FREE · LOW FAT · LOW FIBER · LOW FODMAP

Étouffée is a classic dish in both Cajun and Creole cuisines, both of which originated in Louisiana. It shares a flavor profile with gumbo and jambalaya, but features a lighter blond sauce, made with chicken stock in this recipe.

2 cups water

1 cup white rice

2 tablespoons onion- or
  shallot-infused olive oil

2 celery stalks, chopped

1 green bell pepper, peeled
  and chopped

1 cup plus 2 tablespoons
  chicken stock, divided

1 tablespoon cornstarch

1. In a medium saucepan over high heat, bring the water and rice to a boil. Reduce the heat to low, cover the pot, and cook for 15 to 20 minutes, until all the liquid has been absorbed.

2. Meanwhile, in a large pan or skillet over medium heat, heat the olive oil until shimmering.

3. Add the celery and bell pepper and cook for 5 to 10 minutes, until soft.

4. Add the cooked rice to the pan and stir the ingredients together.

5. Add 1 cup of the chicken stock to the pan, and bring to a simmer over medium-high heat for 5 minutes.

6. In a small bowl, whisk together the remaining 2 tablespoons of chicken stock and the cornstarch, creating a thick slurry.

7. While stirring the étouffée, pour the slurry into the pan to thicken the sauce.

8. Remove the pan from the heat. Allow the sauce to sit and thicken for up to 5 minutes, then serve.

ingredient tip: Étouffée often contains shellfish, and shrimp would be an easily digestible, protein-rich addition to this dish. Add in shrimp during the last 5 minutes of cook time.

Per Serving: Calories: 189; Total Fat: 1g; Saturated Fat: 0g; Total Carbohydrates: 41g; Fiber: 2g; Sugars: 1; Protein: 4g

Jambalaya

PREP TIME 15 MINUTES ⁂ COOK TIME 30 MINUTES ⁂ SERVES 2 TO 4

FLARE-UP · REMISSION · DAIRY-FREE · GLUTEN-FREE · LOW FAT · LOW FIBER · LOW FODMAP

Jambalaya is a Louisiana Cajun dish that is similar to Spanish paella. Traditionally, it features the so-called holy trinity (onion, celery, and green bell pepper), a spicy tomato base, and a variety of meats. This version is completely Crohn's-friendly, made gentle enough for a flare-up.

2 cups water

1 cup white rice

2 tablespoons onion- or shallot-infused olive oil

2 celery stalks, chopped

1 green bell pepper, peeled and chopped

2 bay leaves

½ cup tomato sauce

2 tablespoons tomato paste

¼ teaspoon ground thyme

1. In a medium saucepan over high heat, bring the water and rice to a boil. Reduce the heat to low, cover the pot, and cook for 15 to 20 minutes, until all the water has been absorbed.

2. Meanwhile, in a large skillet over medium heat, heat the olive oil until shimmering.

3. Add the celery, bell pepper, and bay leaves to the pan and cook for 5 to 10 minutes, until soft.

4. Add the cooked rice to the pan and stir.

5. Add the tomato sauce, tomato paste, and thyme to the pan and simmer for 10 minutes.

6. Remove the bay leaves and serve.

ingredient tip: Shrimp or chicken goes well in this dish, if you would like to add meat. You can add shredded cooked chicken in step 5, or cook bite-size pieces of raw chicken with the vegetables in step 3. Whether the shrimp are raw or cooked, you can add them in step 5 as well.

Per Serving: Calories: 251; Total Fat: 7g; Saturated Fat: 1g; Total Carbohydrates: 42g; Fiber: 2g; Sugars: 3g; Protein: 4g

Paella

PREP TIME 15 MINUTES ✹ COOK TIME 30 MINUTES ✹ SERVES 2 TO 4

FLARE-UP · REMISSION · DAIRY-FREE · GLUTEN-FREE · LOW FAT · LOW FIBER · LOW FODMAP

A one-pan dish, traditional paella contains rice, olive oil, saffron, and a variety of vegetables or meats. Spanish flavors are about to make a wonderful addition to your meal repertoire!

2 tablespoons garlic-infused olive oil
1 red bell pepper, peeled and chopped

1 (15-ounce) can diced tomatoes with their juices
8 ounces mushrooms, sliced
1 zucchini, peeled, seeded, and chopped

3 cups vegetable stock
½ teaspoon ground turmeric
1 cup white rice
8 pitted green olives, sliced
Lemon juice

1. In a large Dutch oven or deep skillet, heat the olive oil over medium heat until shimmering.

2. Add the bell pepper, tomatoes with their juices, mushrooms, and zucchini and cook for 5 minutes, until soft.

3. Add the stock and turmeric, increase the heat to medium-high, and bring the mixture to a boil.

4. Add the rice, reduce the heat to medium-low, cover, and cook for 15 to 20 minutes, until the rice is fully cooked.

5. Serve with sliced green olives and a squeeze of lemon juice.

ingredient tip: Saffron, which is traditionally used to color and flavor paella, is expensive and can be hard to find. This recipe uses turmeric, a mild-flavored spice with the same magical yellow hue, but you could also use a few threads of saffron if you have it.

Per Serving: Calories: 297; Total Fat: 9g; Saturated Fat: 1g; Total Carbohydrates: 48g; Fiber: 4g; Sugars: 7g; Protein: 7g

Pasta with Avocado Pesto

PREP TIME 5 MINUTES ※ COOK TIME 15 MINUTES ※ SERVES 2 TO 4

FLARE-UP · REMISSION · DAIRY-FREE · LOW FIBER · LOW FODMAP

Pesto is an Italian sauce traditionally made with olive oil, pine nuts, garlic, salt, basil, and Parmesan cheese. Here, it has been modified for dairy-free and nut-free diets, but it still has the sumptuous, rich flavor of pesto.

- 2 quarts plus 2 tablespoons water, divided
- 8 ounces pasta, any shape
- 1 avocado, diced
- 1 tablespoon garlic-infused olive oil
- 1 cup fresh basil
- 2 tablespoons lemon juice
- ¼ teaspoon salt

1. In a large stockpot over high heat, bring 2 quarts of water to a boil.
2. Add the pasta and cook for 8 to 12 minutes, until tender.
3. Meanwhile, combine the avocado, olive oil, basil, lemon juice, 2 tablespoons of water, and salt in a blender or food processor and pulse or puree until the pesto reaches your desired texture—you might prefer it totally smooth or with a little texture.
4. Drain the pasta.
5. Add the pesto to the pasta and stir until the pasta is evenly coated.
6. Serve this pasta as your main meal or as a side dish.

ingredient tip: Pesto can be made by substituting ⅓ cup ground pine nuts and ⅔ cup grated Parmesan cheese for the avocado in step 3, if these do not trigger flare-ups for you.

Per Serving: Calories: 176; Total Fat: 10g; Saturated Fat: 1g; Total Carbohydrates: 21g; Fiber: 5g; Sugars: 1g; Protein: 4g

Pasta with Red Sauce

PREP TIME 5 MINUTES ✕ **COOK TIME** 15 MINUTES ✕ **SERVES** 2 TO 4

FLARE-UP · REMISSION · DAIRY-FREE · LOW FAT · LOW FIBER · LOW FODMAP

This is a meal on frequent rotation in our house. A simple pasta served with Crohn's-friendly marinara sauce is a dish you can eat as is or jazz up any way you like. Why spend $15 or more on spaghetti at a restaurant when you can have something just as good (and good for you) in the comfort of your own home?

2 quarts water

8 ounces dry pasta, any shape

1 (15-ounce) can tomato sauce

1 cup canned diced tomatoes, drained

2 tablespoons garlic-infused olive oil, divided

1 tablespoon Italian seasoning

¼ teaspoon salt

1. In a large stockpot over high heat, bring the water to a boil.

2. Cook the pasta for 8 to 12 minutes, until tender.

3. Meanwhile, in a medium saucepan, combine the tomato sauce, diced tomatoes, 1 tablespoon of garlic-infused olive oil, Italian seasoning, and salt.

4. Cook the sauce over medium-low heat for 10 to 15 minutes, until the pasta is ready.

5. Drain the pasta and drizzle with the remaining tablespoon of oil. Toss the pasta in the sauce until the noodles are coated evenly.

6. Serve with soft bread to mop up the delicious sauce.

substitution: Make this recipe gluten-free by using your favorite gluten-free pasta.

ingredient tip: You can also use this marinara sauce on pizza or meatball subs.

Per Serving: Calories: 186; Total Fat: 8g; Saturated Fat: 1g; Total Carbohydrates: 26g; Fiber: 5g; Sugars: 6g; Protein: 5g

Tomato-Basil Pasta

PREP TIME UNDER 5 MINUTES ✳ **COOK TIME** 15 MINUTES ✳ **SERVES** 2 TO 4

FLARE-UP · REMISSION · DAIRY-FREE · LOW FAT · LOW FIBER · LOW FODMAP

Basil is an antioxidant-rich herb that is pleasantly gentle on your system. It is particularly tasty as prepared here, and it is full of vitamins and minerals. Feel free to liberally add the fresh, slightly sweet flavor of basil to a wide variety of dishes.

2 quarts water

8 ounces angel-hair pasta

1 (15-ounce) can diced
  tomatoes with their juices

1 tablespoon tomato paste

8 fresh basil
  leaves, chopped

2 tablespoons garlic-infused
  olive oil, divided

1. In a large stockpot over high heat, bring the water to a boil.

2. Add the pasta and cook for 8 to 12 minutes, until tender.

3. Meanwhile, in a medium saucepan, combine the tomatoes, tomato paste, basil, and 1 tablespoon of the garlic-infused olive oil.

4. Cook the sauce over medium-low heat for 10 to 15 minutes, until the pasta is ready.

5. Drain the pasta and drizzle with the remaining tablespoon of oil.

6. Toss the pasta in the sauce until the noodles are coated evenly.

7. Serve warm or enjoy cold as a pasta salad on a hot day.

ingredient tip: Any shape of pasta works in this recipe, but angel-hair pasta adds a unique texture that can help add some variety to your meals.

Per Serving: Calories: 172; Total Fat: 8g; Saturated Fat: 1g; Total Carbohydrates: 22g; Fiber: 3g; Sugars: 4g; Protein: 5g

Caprese Pasta

PREP TIME 5 MINUTES ✳ COOK TIME 15 MINUTES ✳ SERVES 4

FLARE-UP · REMISSION · LOW FAT · LOW FIBER · LOW FODMAP

Caprese is a fresh Italian salad, composed of mozzarella, tomato, basil, olive oil, and salt. This recipe has been modified to make it appropriate for a flare-up or remission, and you can choose to omit the mozzarella for an even milder meal.

2 quarts water

12 ounces dry pasta, any shape

1 (15-ounce) can diced tomatoes, drained

2 tablespoons chopped fresh basil

4 ounces fresh or shredded mozzarella (optional)

2 teaspoons balsamic vinegar

3 tablespoons garlic-infused olive oil

Salt

1. In a large stockpot over high heat, bring the water to a boil.

2. Add the pasta and boil for 8 to 12 minutes, until tender.

3. Meanwhile, in a large bowl, combine the tomatoes, basil, mozzarella (if using), balsamic vinegar, and olive oil. (If the mozzarella is fresh, dice or crumble it before adding it to the bowl.)

4. Drain the pasta and add it to the large bowl.

5. Mix the ingredients together and serve with a sprinkling of salt.

substitution: To make this recipe gluten-free, simply use your favorite gluten-free pasta.

Per Serving: Calories: 244; Total Fat: 12g; Saturated Fat: 2g; Total Carbohydrates: 31g; Fiber: 4g; Sugars: 4g; Protein: 6g

Moroccan-Inspired Pasta Bake

**PREP TIME 10 MINUTES ✳ COOK TIME 40 MINUTES, PLUS 10 MINUTES TO REST
SERVES 2 TO 4**

FLARE-UP · REMISSION · DAIRY-FREE · LOW FAT · LOW FIBER · LOW FODMAP

———————————

Morocco is a North African country on the Mediterranean Sea, sitting just below Spain. Their traditional flavors of ginger, cinnamon, cumin, lemon, and tomato are robust and Crohn's-friendly. This pasta bake is inspired by Moroccan tagine, a one-pot meal of meat and vegetables.

8 ounces dry pasta,
  any shape

1 cup pumpkin puree

1 (15-ounce) can diced
  tomatoes with their juices

2 cups chicken stock

½ teaspoon ground ginger

½ teaspoon ground cumin

½ teaspoon ground
  cinnamon

½ teaspoon salt

½ cup panko bread crumbs

1 tablespoon olive oil

1. Preheat the oven to 425°F.
2. In a large bowl, combine the dry pasta, pumpkin, diced tomatoes with their juices, stock, ginger, cumin, cinnamon, and salt. Mix until all the ingredients are evenly distributed.
3. Fill a 9-by-9-inch baking dish with the pasta mixture.
4. Cover the dish with a double layer of foil, and bake for 30 minutes.
5. Meanwhile, in a small bowl, mix the panko and olive oil together.
6. Remove the foil, sprinkle the panko on top of the pasta, and bake, uncovered, for 10 more minutes.
7. Remove from the oven and allow to rest and thicken for 10 minutes. Serve warm.

substitution: Make this recipe gluten-free by using your favorite gluten-free pasta and leaving out the panko.

———————————

Per Serving: Calories: 230; Total Fat: 6g; Saturated Fat: 1g; Total Carbohydrates: 37g; Fiber: 6g; Sugars: 7g; Protein: 9g

Mushroom Pasta

PREP TIME 10 MINUTES ※ **COOK TIME** 15 MINUTES ※ **SERVES** 2 TO 4

FLARE-UP · REMISSION · DAIRY-FREE · LOW FAT · LOW FIBER · LOW FODMAP

This recipe will satisfy any craving for a creamy, luscious sauce—without any dairy. Cream sauces can sit heavily on your system, but this one is light and easy to digest. Enjoy this mushroom pasta as a main dish or a side.

1 quart water

8 ounces dry pasta, any shape

2 tablespoons garlic-infused olive oil

1 tablespoon flour

1 cup unsweetened plain nondairy milk

8 ounces mushrooms, sliced

1 tablespoon lemon juice

¼ teaspoon ground thyme

¼ teaspoon salt

1 tablespoon chopped fresh parsley, for garnish

1. In a medium stockpot, bring the water and pasta to a boil over high heat.

2. Cook for 8 to 12 minutes, until tender. Drain.

3. Meanwhile, in a small pan over medium heat, heat the garlic-infused olive oil until shimmering.

4. Stir in the flour to form a roux, and cook for 1 to 2 minutes, until the mixture starts to turn golden brown.

5. Adding ¼ cup at a time, stir in the nondairy milk to make a thick sauce.

6. Add the mushrooms, lemon juice, thyme, and salt; mix well. Cook for 2 to 3 minutes, until the mushrooms are cooked through.

7. Serve each plate of pasta with a heaping spoonful of mushroom sauce and a sprinkling of fresh parsley.

ingredient tip: Any type of mushroom is suitable for this dish, but you might find that you have a preference. Experiment with button, cremini, chanterelle, shiitake, oyster, or portabella mushrooms.

Per Serving: Calories: 237; Total Fat: 16g; Saturated Fat: 2g; Total Carbohydrates: 21g; Fiber: 3g; Sugars: 2g; Protein: 6g

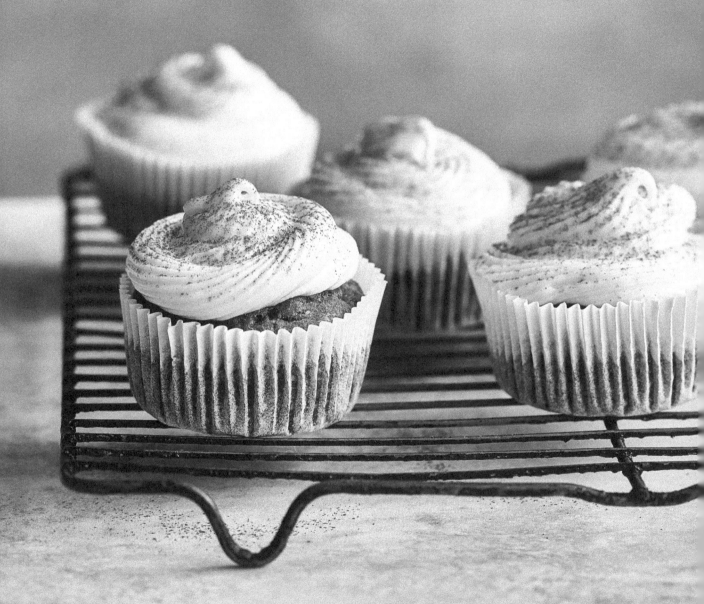

Banana Cupcakes · *page 171*

CHAPTER 11

Desserts

After cooking your way through this book, you are surely ready for a decadent treat. Each of these ten desserts are dairy-free, and more than half are gluten-free! Enjoy these freely when you need something sweet and don't want to worry about whether it will suit your digestive system.

Watermelon Sorbet

PREP TIME 5 MINUTES ✳ **SERVES** 4

FLARE-UP · REMISSION · DAIRY-FREE · GLUTEN-FREE · LOW FAT · LOW FIBER · LOW FODMAP · PALEO

This sorbet is like biting into a fresh slice of watermelon on a hot summer day, but even better. Watermelons are not always in season, so try buying them when they are available, dicing them, and freezing the cubes in freezer-safe containers for year-round use.

2 cups chopped seedless watermelon

2 cups ice

1 tablespoon lime juice

¼ teaspoon salt

1. Put all the ingredients in a blender and blend on high for 30 to 60 seconds, until smooth.
2. Serve immediately or freeze.

substitution: Try this sorbet with different melons, like cantaloupe or honeydew.

make ahead: You can make large batches of sorbet to keep in the freezer for up to 1 month.

Per Serving: Calories: 16; Total Fat: 0g; Saturated Fat: 0g; Total Carbohydrates: 4g; Fiber: 0g; Sugars: 3g; Protein: 0g

Ginger-Peach Sorbet

PREP TIME 5 MINUTES ✳ **SERVES** 4

FLARE-UP · REMISSION · DAIRY-FREE · GLUTEN-FREE · LOW FAT · LOW FIBER · LOW FODMAP · PALEO

The beautiful thing about sorbet is that it isn't just a dairy-free alternative to ice cream—it's also essentially a frozen smoothie you eat with a spoon. You can make any smoothie into a frozen dessert by simply decreasing the liquid.

2 cups frozen chopped peaches

2 bananas, peeled

1 teaspoon ground ginger

1. Put all the ingredients in a blender or food processor and blend on high for 30 to 60 seconds, until smooth.
2. Serve immediately or freeze.

make ahead: You can make large batches of sorbet to keep in the freezer for a refreshing and nutritious treat.

Per Serving: Calories: 113; Total Fat: 1g; Saturated Fat: 0g; Total Carbohydrates: 28g; Fiber: 4g; Sugars: 20g; Protein: 2g

Poached Pears

PREP TIME 15 MINUTES ✳ **COOK TIME** 20 MINUTES, PLUS 10 MINUTES TO COOL ✳ **SERVES** 4

FLARE-UP · REMISSION · DAIRY-FREE · GLUTEN-FREE · LOW FAT · LOW FIBER · PALEO

This fruity dessert has the added benefits of anti-inflammatory agents like cinnamon and ginger. The spices dampen the sweetness of the pears, but don't worry, they are still pleasantly sweet.

4 cups water

1 teaspoon vanilla extract

¼ cup sugar

1 teaspoon ground cinnamon

1 teaspoon ground ginger

4 pears, peeled, halved, and cored

1. In a large saucepan over medium-high heat, combine the water, vanilla, sugar, cinnamon, and ginger.
2. Bring the liquid to a boil.
3. Reduce the heat to medium low and add the pear halves.
4. Cook for 10 minutes, flip the pear halves, and cook for 10 more minutes.
5. Remove the pan from the heat and let the pears cool in the liquid for 5 to 10 minutes.
6. Serve with a drizzle of the poaching liquid.

ingredient tip: The most common pears at the supermarket are Anjou, Bartlett, and Bosc. Bartlett pears are the softest, sweetest, and juiciest. Bosc pears are crisp and mildly sweet. Anjou pears are somewhere in between. Any variety works well in this recipe.

Per Serving: Calories: 156; Total Fat: 0g; Saturated Fat: 0g; Total Carbohydrates: 41g; Fiber: 6g; Sugars: 30g; Protein: 1g

Banana Pudding

PREP TIME 5 MINUTES, PLUS 3 HOURS TO CHILL ※ COOK TIME 10 MINUTES ※ SERVES 4

FLARE-UP · REMISSION · DAIRY-FREE · GLUTEN-FREE · LOW FIBER · LOW FODMAP · LOW FAT · PALEO

Pudding would be extremely gentle on your gut, if only it were dairy-free. Well, you are in luck! This banana pudding is completely dairy-free and still creamy and luscious.

½ cup sugar

3 tablespoons cornstarch

Pinch salt

2 bananas, divided

2 cups unsweetened plain nondairy milk

1 teaspoon vanilla extract

1. In a small bowl, whisk together the sugar, cornstarch, and salt.
2. In a large bowl, mash 1 banana until few lumps remain. Whisk in the nondairy milk and vanilla.
3. In a medium saucepan, combine the wet and dry ingredients, whisking them together until there are no lumps.
4. Cook the pudding over low heat for 5 to 10 minutes, until thickened. Stir occasionally to prevent burning.
5. Pour the pudding into a bowl or into individual serving dishes, transfer it to the refrigerator, and let it chill for 3 hours.
6. Slice the remaining banana, and place the slices on top of the pudding before serving.

substitution: This pudding is a simple base that you can modify to your tastes. For vanilla pudding, omit the banana and double the vanilla (or use vanilla-flavored nondairy milk). For chocolate pudding, add 1 teaspoon cocoa powder. Top the pudding with jam or jelly of any flavor. Substitute the banana with avocado for a healthy-fat-filled pudding.

Per Serving: Calories: 193; Total Fat: 2g; Saturated Fat: 0g; Total Carbohydrates: 45g; Fiber: 2g; Sugars: 32g; Protein: 1g

Rice Pudding

PREP TIME 5 MINUTES ※ **COOK TIME** 45 MINUTES ※ **SERVES** 4

FLARE-UP · REMISSION · DAIRY-FREE · GLUTEN-FREE · LOW FAT · LOW FIBER · LOW FODMAP

In the United States, we tend to think of rice as being a side dish, but in many parts of the world, it is used at every meal, including dessert. As a blank canvas, rice pudding can take on any flavor you choose. Here, it has a subtle but pleasing vanilla taste to complement the decadent texture.

2 cups water

1 cup white rice

2 cups unsweetened plain nondairy milk, divided

1 teaspoon vanilla extract

¼ cup sugar

¼ teaspoon salt

1 egg

1. In a medium saucepan over high heat, bring the water and rice to a boil. Reduce the heat to low, cover, and cook for 15 to 20 minutes, until the rice can be fluffed with a fork.

2. Add the nondairy milk, vanilla, sugar, and salt to the cooked rice and stir together over medium heat.

3. Cook for 15 minutes, stirring occasionally.

4. Using a cup or ladle, scoop about ½ cup of hot liquid out of the saucepan. In a small bowl, beat the egg, and then slowly whisk the hot milk into the egg. This step will help prevent the egg from scrambling when you add it to the pudding.

5. Slowly stir the egg mixture into the pudding and cook for 5 minutes more.

6. Serve warm.

substitution: This is a basic rice pudding recipe. Feel free to jazz it up with spices like cinnamon or ginger, make it rich with cocoa powder, or lighten it with fruit.

Per Serving: Calories: 255; Total Fat: 3g; Saturated Fat: 0g; Total Carbohydrates: 50g; Fiber: 1g; Sugars: 13g; Protein: 5g

Cereal Bars

PREP TIME 5 MINUTES ⊗ **COOK TIME** 10 MINUTES, PLUS 10 MINUTES TO COOL
MAKES 12 BARS

FLARE-UP · REMISSION · DAIRY-FREE · LOW FAT · LOW FIBER · LOW FODMAP

The key to these cereal bars is their low fiber content. Choosing easy-to-digest cereal makes this dessert a great way to finish out your final meal of the day. Examples of low-fiber cereals include Rice Krispies, Corn Flakes, Apple Jacks, Cocoa Krispies, Fruity Pebbles, Chex, Kix, and Trix—all are of which are delicious in this recipe.

3 tablespoons vegetable or canola oil

10 to 12 ounces marshmallows, any size

6 cups dry cereal

1. Line a 9-by-13-inch baking dish with parchment paper.
2. In a large stockpot, warm the oil over low heat.
3. Add the marshmallows to the pot and melt them down. Stir frequently to prevent burning.
4. Remove the pot from the heat and stir in the cereal.
5. Transfer the cereal-marshmallow mixture to the prepared baking dish, and press it down into all the corners so the bars will have a flat top.
6. Let the bars cool for 5 to 10 minutes, then cut them into 2-inch squares.

substitution: Make this recipe gluten-free by choosing your favorite gluten-free cereal.

make it easier: You can purchase marshmallow fluff instead of melting down the marshmallows, which would make the process a little faster.

make ahead: You can make pans of these treats ahead of time and store the bars in freezer bags, separated with wax paper, for up to 90 days.

Per Serving: Calories: 156; Total Fat: 4g; Saturated Fat: 0g; Total Carbohydrates: 31g; Fiber: 0g; Sugars: 15g; Protein: 1g

Oatmeal Cookies

PREP TIME 15 MINUTES ⁕ **COOK TIME** 10 MINUTES, PLUS 10 MINUTES TO REST
MAKES 12 COOKIES

FLARE-UP · REMISSION · DAIRY-FREE · LOW FAT · LOW FIBER · LOW FODMAP

There is something so comforting about an oatmeal cookie. This recipe omits the perpetually maligned raisins for a classic, chewy, and not-too-sweet oatmeal cookie that is gentle on the system.

½ cup all-purpose flour
¼ cup sugar
½ teaspoon baking soda
1 teaspoon ground cinnamon

1 cup rolled oats
¼ cup vegetable or
  canola oil

¼ cup unsweetened
  applesauce
1 teaspoon vanilla extract

1. Preheat the oven to 375°F. Line a baking sheet with parchment paper.
2. In a large bowl, whisk together the flour, sugar, baking soda, and cinnamon.
3. Add the oats, oil, applesauce, and vanilla, mixing until the oats are evenly coated.
4. Scoop out 2 tablespoons of the batter, roll it into a ball, and lightly press it flat onto the prepared baking sheet. Repeat 12 times, spacing the cookies at least 1 inch apart.
5. Bake for 10 minutes or until the cookies are golden brown.
6. Allow the cookies to rest on the baking sheet for 5 to 10 minutes to firm up.
7. Serve warm, or store in an airtight container at room temperature for up to 3 days or in the freezer for 2 to 3 weeks.

make ahead: Leftover cookies make a nice breakfast on the go.

Per Serving: Calories: 104; Total Fat: 5g; Saturated Fat: 0g; Total Carbohydrates: 13g; Fiber: 1g; Sugars: 5g; Protein: 2g

Peanut Butter Cookies

PREP TIME 10 MINUTES ✻ **COOK TIME** 10 MINUTES
MAKES 2 **DOZEN COOKIES**

FLARE-UP · REMISSION · DAIRY-FREE · LOW FIBER · LOW FODMAP

What if your dessert provided some protein? Thank goodness for peanut butter cookies. Creamy peanut butter is considered low-fiber and low-residue, but is a good source of protein and other essential nutrients.

1 cup all-purpose flour

1 cup sugar

1 teaspoon baking soda

¼ teaspoon salt

1 cup natural creamy
   peanut butter

⅓ cup unsweetened plain
   nondairy milk

1 teaspoon vanilla extract

1. Preheat the oven to 350°F. Line a baking sheet with parchment paper.
2. In a large bowl, whisk together the flour, sugar, baking soda, and salt.
3. In a medium bowl, stir together the peanut butter, nondairy milk, and vanilla.
4. Add the wet ingredients to the dry ingredients and mix with clean or gloved hands. The dough will be too stiff for a spoon.
5. Knead the dough until there are no patches of dry ingredients remaining.
6. Use a tablespoon or a 1-tablespoon cookie scoop to make 24 balls, and place them on the prepared baking sheet at least 1 inch apart.
7. Using the back of a fork, flatten each ball in a crisscross pattern.
8. Bake for 10 minutes for chewy cookies, 12 to 13 minutes for crispier cookies.
9. Serve warm or cooled.

substitution: You can make these cookies with sunflower seed butter for a peanut-free option.

make ahead: These cookies freeze well for up to 60 days.

Per Serving (1 cookie): Calories: 118; Total Fat: 6g; Saturated Fat: 1g; Total Carbohydrates: 14g; Fiber: 2g; Sugars: 9g; Protein: 3g

Berry Crumble

PREP TIME 10 **MINUTES** ※ **COOK TIME** 25 **MINUTES** ※ **SERVES** 9

REMISSION · DAIRY-FREE · LOW FAT · LOW FODMAP

Oats are a naturally gluten-free, protein-rich whole grain. They are easy to digest and full of fiber, vitamins, minerals, and antioxidants called avenanthramides. The berry skins in this recipe increase the fiber content, but the cooking process softens them significantly.

3 cups blueberries
3 cups sliced strawberries
1 tablespoon lime juice
2 tablespoons cornstarch
1 cup rolled oats
1 teaspoon ground cinnamon
¼ cup vegetable or canola oil
¼ cup honey

1. Preheat the oven to 375°F.
2. In a medium bowl, combine the blueberries, strawberries, lime juice, and cornstarch. Mix well until there are no lumps of cornstarch.
3. Fill a 9-by-9-inch baking dish with the berry mixture.
4. In a separate medium bowl, combine the oats, cinnamon, oil, and honey. Mix until all ingredients are evenly distributed.
5. Cover the berry mixture with the oat topping.
6. Bake for 35 to 40 minutes, until the top is golden brown and crisp.
7. Serve warm.

make it milder: You can substitute peeled peaches or nectarines for the berries to make a dessert more suitable for a flare-up.

Per Serving: Calories: 169; Total Fat: 7g; Saturated Fat: 1g; Total Carbohydrates: 27g; Fiber: 3g; Sugars: 15g; Protein: 2g

Banana Cupcakes

PREP TIME 20 MINUTES ※ COOK TIME 30 MINUTES, PLUS 30 MINUTES TO COOL
MAKES 1 DOZEN CUPCAKES

FLARE-UP · REMISSION · DAIRY-FREE · LOW FAT · LOW FIBER · LOW FODMAP

This recipe is modified from the banana bread I bake for my family on a regular basis. It is moist with a tender crumb, and not too sweet—although it's still sure to satisfy your sweet tooth.

For the cupcakes
1¼ cups all-purpose flour
⅔ cup sugar
1 teaspoon baking soda

1 teaspoon ground cinnamon
3 ripe bananas
½ cup vegetable or
   canola oil
½ cup nondairy milk
2 teaspoons vanilla extract

For the frosting
3 cups powdered sugar
2½ tablespoons
   vegan butter
3 tablespoons nondairy milk
2 teaspoons vanilla extract

To make the cupcakes

1. Preheat the oven to 375°F. Line a 12-well cupcake tin with cupcake liners, or coat with nonstick cooking spray.

2. In a large bowl, whisk together the flour, sugar, baking soda, and cinnamon.

3. In a separate large bowl, mash the bananas with a fork or potato masher until few or no lumps remain.

4. Add the oil, nondairy milk, and vanilla to the mashed bananas and mix well.

5. Add the wet ingredients to the dry ingredients and whisk together thoroughly.

6. Fill each well of the cupcake tin with ¼ to ⅓ cup of batter until all the batter has been used and all the wells are filled.

continued...

Banana Cupcakes *continued*

7. Bake for 30 minutes, watching during the last 10 minutes to prevent over-cooking. The cupcakes are done when a toothpick inserted into the center comes out clean.

8. Allow the cupcakes 20 to 30 minutes to cool.

To make the frosting

9. In a large bowl, combine the powdered sugar, vegan butter, nondairy milk, and vanilla.

10. Using an electric mixer, or a whisk and a lot of muscle, blend the ingredients together until the icing is smooth and spreadable.

11. Frost the cupcakes and serve.

make ahead: These cupcakes make a great grab-and-go breakfast. You can even omit the frosting and dust them with powdered sugar to make them a little less sweet.

Per Serving: Calories: 200; Total Fat: 10g; Saturated Fat: 1g; Total Carbohydrates: 27g; Fiber: 2g; Sugars: 15g; Protein: 2g

Food Reaction Tracker

Your doctor or dietitian may recommend that you reintroduce foods into your diet during remission, to test which foods are triggers for you. A food diary is a helpful tool for recording how individual foods affect you.

Reintroduce foods one at a time, one every few days, to track symptoms accurately. Reintroducing more than one food at a time can make it difficult to determine which food caused a reaction.

	FOODS EATEN	BOWEL MOVEMENT?	ABDOMINAL PAIN (1–10)	FLARE-UP?
SUN				
MON				
TUE				
WED				
THUR				
FRI				
SAT				

You may want to start with a safe food and then add in a similar but potentially more troublesome food. For example, if you know white rice works well, you could try adding brown rice. You could also try a safe fruit with the skin on, or try it less thoroughly cooked.

Working with a dietitian can remove a lot of the guesswork, since they can partner with you every step of the way.

STRESS & EMOTIONS	NAUSEA? VOMITING? DIARRHEA? CONSTIPATION?	OTHER NOTES

Measurement Conversions

Volume Equivalents	US STANDARD	U.S. STANDARD (OUNCES)	METRIC (APPROXIMATE)
Liquid	2 tablespoons	1 fl. oz.	30 mL
	¼ cup	2 fl. oz.	60 mL
	½ cup	4 fl. oz.	120 mL
	1 cup	8 fl. oz.	240 mL
	1½ cups	12 fl. oz.	355 mL
	2 cups or 1 pint	16 fl. oz.	475 mL
	4 cups or 1 quart	32 fl. oz.	1 L
	1 gallon	128 fl. oz.	4 L
Dry	⅛ teaspoon	—	0.5 mL
	¼ teaspoon	—	1 mL
	½ teaspoon	—	2 mL
	¾ teaspoon	—	4 mL
	1 teaspoon	—	5 mL
	1 tablespoon	—	15 mL
	¼ cup	—	59 mL
	⅓ cup	—	79 mL
	½ cup	—	118 mL
	⅔ cup	—	156 mL
	¾ cup	—	177 mL
	1 cup	—	235 mL
	2 cups or 1 pint	—	475 mL
	3 cups	—	700 mL
	4 cups or 1 quart	—	1 L
	½ gallon	—	2 L
	1 gallon	—	4 L

Oven Temperatures

FAHRENHEIT	CELSIUS (APPROXIMATE)
250°F	120°C
300°F	150°C
325°F	165°C
350°F	180°C
375°F	190°C
400°F	200°C
425°F	220°C
450°F	230°C

Weight Equivalents

U.S. STANDARD	METRIC (APPROXIMATE)
½ ounce	15 g
1 ounce	30 g
2 ounces	60 g
4 ounces	115 g
8 ounces	225 g
12 ounces	340 g
16 ounces or 1 pound	455 g

Resources

Academy of Nutrition and Dietetics: Find an Expert
EatRight.org/find-an-expert

American College of Gastroenterology
GI.org

American Gastroenterological Association
Gastro.org

Crohnology
Crohnology.com

Crohn's & Colitis Community
CrohnsColitisCommunity.org

Crohn's & Colitis Foundation
CrohnsColitisFoundation.org

Healthline: Crohn's Nutrition Guide
Healthline.com/health/crohns-disease/nutrition-guide

Intense Intestines Foundation
Facebook.com/pg/IntenseIntestines/about/?ref=page_internal

Monash University: FODMAP resources
MonashFODMAP.com/about-fodmap-and-ibs/fodmap
-diet-resources

References

Carreon, David, and Jessica A. Gold. "The Mind-Gut Connection: What Is it and How Did It Evolve?" Published February 21, 2018. PsychiatricTimes.com/neuropsychiatry /mind-gut-connection-what-it-and-how-did-it-evolve.

Cherney, Kristeen. "Crohn's Nutrition Guide." Reviewed June 26, 2018. Healthline.com /health/crohns-disease/nutrition-guide.

Crohn's & Colitis (website). Accessed February 29, 2020. CrohnsandColitis.com.

Crohn's & Colitis (website). "Ulcerative Colitis Nutrition & Exercise." Accessed February 29, 2020. CrohnsandColitis.com/living-with-crohns-uc/ulcerative-colitis /diet-and-exercise?cid=ppc_ppd_ggl_uc_da_ulcerative_colitis_diet_Exact_64Z1867746 &gclid=EAIaIQobChMI5qSZ5sfI5wIVysDACh1ysg8MEAAYAiAAEgLqi_D_BwE.

Crohn's & Colitis Foundation (website). Accessed February 29, 2020. CrohnsColitisFoundation.org.

Crohn's & Colitis Foundation (website). "Diet and Nutrition." Accessed February 29, 2020. CrohnsColitisFoundation.org/diet-and-nutrition.

Crohn's & Colitis Foundation (website). "Signs and Symptoms of Ulcerative Colitis." Accessed February 29. 2020. CrohnsColitisFoundation.org/what-is-ulcerative-colitis /symptoms.

Dennett, Carrie. "Digestive Wellness: Crohn's Disease." Published December 2016. TodaysDietitian.com/newarchives/1216p12.shtml.

Donnellan, Clare F., Lee H. Yann, and Simon Lal. "Nutritional Management of Crohn's Disease." *Therapeutic Advances in Gastroenterology* 6, no. 3 (May 2013): 231–242. Doi: 10.1177/1756283X13577715.

Fine, Allison. "Managing Stress Through Mindfulness." Center for Chronic Illness. Accessed February 29. 2020. online.crohnscolitisfoundation.org /site/DocServer/CCFA_April_2018_Mindfullness_and_Stress_Presentation _PDF.pdf;jsessionid=00000000.app30130a?docID=34307&NONCE _TOKEN=9434AAE7F45A07B02DEA87446C4E5FA0.

Garson, Philippa. "7 Breakfast Recipes for People with Crohn's." Updated August 8, 2018. EverydayHealth.com/crohns-disease/diet/breakfast-recipes-people-with -crohns.

Harvard Medical School (website). "The Gut-Brain Connection." Accessed February 29, 2020 Health.Harvard.edu/diseases-and-conditions/the-gut-brain-connection.

Hayden, Natalie. "Breakfast with IBD: What 6 Morning Meals Look Like." Accessed February 29, 2020. OshiHealth.com/breakfast-with-ibd-what-6-morning-meals -look-like.

IBS Diets (website). "FODMAP Food List." Updated March 18, 2020. IBSDiets.org /fodmap-diet/fodmap-food-list.

John Hopkins Medicine (website). "The Brain-Gut Connection." Accessed February 29, 2020. HopkinsMedicine.org/health/wellness-and-prevention/the-brain-gut -connection.

Jones, M. P., J. B. Dilley, D. Drossman, and M. D. Crowell. "Brain-Gut Connections in Functional GI Disorders." *Neurogastroenterology & Motility* 18, no. 2 (January 17, 2006). Doi: 10.1111/j.1365-2982.2005.00730.x.

Kennedy, Kelly. "8 Things to Ask Your Dietitian When Diagnosed with Crohn's Disease." Accessed February 29, 2020. EverydayHealth.com/crohns-disease/diet /things-to-ask-your-dietitian-with-crohns-disease.

Langorst, Jost, H. Wulfert, R. Lauche, et al. "Systematic Review of Complementary and Alternative Medicine Treatments in Inflammatory Bowel Diseases." *Journal of Crohn's and Colitis* 9, no. 1 (December 4, 2014): 86–106. Doi: 10.1093/ecco-jcc/jju007.

Littrell, J. "The Mind-Body Connection: Not Just a Theory Anymore." *Social Work in Health Care* 46, no. 4 (2008): 17–37. Doi: 10.1300/j010v46n04_02.

McCaffrey, Ruth, Terri Frock, and Heidi Garguilo. "Understanding Chronic Pain and the Mind-Body Connection." *Holistic Nurse Practice.* 17, no. 6 (November-December 2003): 281–289.

Nalibof, Bruce D., Michael P. Frese, and Rapgay Lobsang. "Mind/Body Psychological Treatments for Irritable Bowel Syndrome." *Evidence-Based Complementary and Alternative Medicine* 5 (2008). Doi: 10.1093/ecam/nem046.

National Institute of Diabetes and Digestive and Kidney Diseases. "Eating, Diet, & Nutrition for Crohn's Disease." Published September 2017. niddk.nih.gov/health -information/digestive-diseases/crohns-disease/eating-diet-nutrition.

Smith, Melissa M., and Janet L. Bryant. "Mind-Body and Mind-Gut Connection in Inflammatory Bowel Disease." *Gastroenterology Nursing* 25, no. 5 (September–October 2002): 213–217.

Talcott, Susanne. "Study Shows Mango Consumption Has Positive Impact on Inflammatory Bowel Disease." *Texas A&M University*. Published July 31, 2017. MedicalXpress.com/news/2017-07-mango-consumption-positive-impact-inflammatory.html.

Theobald, Mikel. "What to Eat for Crohn's Disease: Tips From a Registered Dietitian." Accessed February 29, 2020. EverydayHealth.com/hs/crohns-disease-treatment-management/what-to-eat-dietitian-tips.

Torres, Joanna, Ellul, Jost Langorst, et al. "European Crohn's and Colitis Organisation Topical Review on Complementary Medicine and Psychotherapy in Inflammatory Bowel Disease. *Journal of Crohn's and Colitis* 13, no. 6 (March 1, 2019): 673–685e. Doi: 10.1093/ecco-jcc/jjz051.

University of Michigan (website). "Mind-Body Wellness." Accessed February 29, 2020. UofMHealth.org/health-library/mente.

Zibdeh, Nour. "Crohn's Disease and Diet." Published September 11, 2019. EatRight.org/health/wellness/digestive-health/crohns-disease-and-diet.

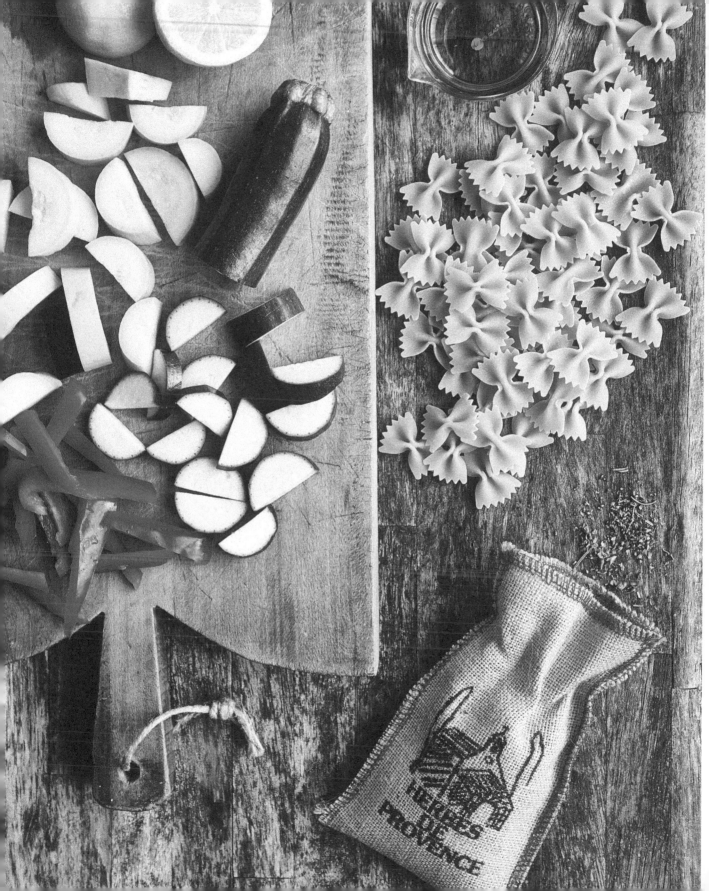

Index

Page locators in **bold** indicate pictures

W

Acknowledgments

Thank you to my husband and my daughter, for giving me the time to follow my dreams.

Thank you to my parents for your bottomless support and babysitting.

Last, but certainly not least, thank you to the wonderful team at Callisto, for all your hard work. It has been an absolute pleasure working with you all.

About the Author

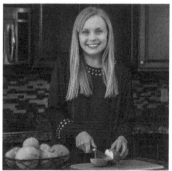

Amanda Foote, RD, is a registered dietitian, author, proud fire wife, and mother. She runs her own virtual nutrition practice, Amanda Foote Nutrition, specializing in food allergies and intolerance, as well as special (therapeutic) diets for medical conditions that require following a specific diet. It is her calling to ensure that food remains an enjoyable, nourishing part of the human experience, despite dietary restrictions.

In addition to her practice, Amanda has worked as a registered dietitian for InnovAge and South Adams County Fire Department. She has a bachelor's degree in dietetics from the University of Northern Colorado, and a bachelor's degree in applied psychology from Regis University.

Amanda lives in Colorado with her family and pets. In her spare time, she enjoys developing new recipes, sketching, crafting, reading, running 5Ks, and all things Disney.

Printed in the USA
CPSIA information can be obtained
at www.ICGtesting.com
CBHW042353200124
3539CB00002B/19